Janet Carolina Negrón Espadas
Aurora Sierra Canto

Nursing and occupational hazards

Janet Carolina Negrón Espadas
Aurora Sierra Canto

Nursing and occupational hazards

Ethical and legal context

ScienciaScripts

Imprint
Any brand names and product names mentioned in this book are subject to trademark, brand or patent protection and are trademarks or registered trademarks of their respective holders. The use of brand names, product names, common names, trade names, product descriptions etc. even without a particular marking in this work is in no way to be construed to mean that such names may be regarded as unrestricted in respect of trademark and brand protection legislation and could thus be used by anyone.

Cover image: www.ingimage.com

This book is a translation from the original published under ISBN 978-3-639-60262-3.

Publisher:
Sciencia Scripts
is a trademark of
Dodo Books Indian Ocean Ltd. and OmniScriptum S.R.L publishing group

120 High Road, East Finchley, London, N2 9ED, United Kingdom
Str. Armeneasca 28/1, office 1, Chisinau MD-2012, Republic of Moldova, Europe
Printed at: see last page
ISBN: 978-620-6-12948-6

Copyright © Janet Carolina Negrón Espadas, Aurora Sierra Canto
Copyright © 2023 Dodo Books Indian Ocean Ltd. and OmniScriptum S.R.L publishing group

INTRODUCTION

At present, various international and national organizations are seeking to create healthy work environments, since the health, safety and well-being of workers are of fundamental importance for the workers themselves and their families, and also for the productivity, competitiveness and sustainability of companies and, therefore, for the economies of countries and the world, according to the World Health Organization (WHO).According to the International Labor Organization (ILO), more than 2 million people die each year as a result of work-related accidents or illnesses. According to conservative estimates, there are 270 million accidents at work and 160 million cases of occupational diseases.Developing countries pay a particularly high price in deaths and injuries, as most people are employed in hazardous activities. This book addresses and analyzes important issues regarding occupational health in general and specifically in health care workers. It is organized in two sections, the first one called **Occupational Risks** and the second one called **Ethical and Legal Context.**

The section on occupational hazards includes six chapters that deal with protection, promotion and prevention of occupational health, as well as the work context of nursing professionals in times of COVID 19.Chapter one, Protection, promotion and prevention of occupational health, conceptualizes the terms related to occupational health, focusing on the first level of care to generate favorable environments, development of personal skills and reorientation of health services, to identify and classify occupational risks, as well as historical data for the creation of agencies for the protection of occupational health. To follow up on the previous chapter, chapter two is presented: Occupational Risks, in which the elements for preparing an occupational health diagnosis are visualized, starting with risk assessment, identification and classification, which allows the variables to be crossed in order to issue a risk report.In this same sense, chapter three: Detection of risks and working conditions, analyzes the changes, environmental conditions and the development of regulatory regulations and adaptations derived from the health contingency by COVID 19 to detect risks and appropriate conditions for the worker in a timely manner.As a follow-up to the previous chapter, chapter four: Network of resources for the efficiency of employee health is presented, which describes the regulatory institutions, regulations and laws that establish strategies for the welfare of workers. It is known that good organization among workers is fundamental, since it favors to encourage employers to guarantee the rights and obligations established by organizations and regulations, as well as access to health services and improve their working conditions to have a better quality of life.Chapter five, entitled Occupational Risks of Health Personnel, focuses mainly on the occupational risks of health personnel, in order to visualize the current problems, the threats, the generation of preventive strategies, as well as to establish the appropriate biosecurity measures that have a direct impact on the vulnerability of health professionals. To conclude this section, chapter six, Labor context in nursing professionals in times of COVID 19 is presented. This chapter analyzes the labor context of nursing professionals since the appearance of the Sars Cov 2 virus, as well as the panorama of the personnel who provided care in the first line against the pandemic. Focused on four aspects, the role, occupational health, mental health and the perception of nursing professionals.

Occupational health professionals have different obligations that include the protection of the life and health of workers, respect for human dignity, the promotion of ethical principles in health policies and programs, and the promotion of the health and safety of workers. occupational. They must also have integrity in professional conduct, impartiality and protection of confidentiality of data on the health and privacy of workers. Therefore, the following section addresses the chapters from this perspective.

Section II. Ethical and legal context, four chapters are included, from seven to ten. This section covers legal aspects, occupational health and safety agencies and nursing actions in health negligence.

Chapter seven: Ethical and legal framework in occupational health, allows the identification of the legal framework that contributes to the establishment of the basic principles, obligations and rights of health workers.

Chapter eight: Psychosocial risk factors in health professionals, presents the classification, impact and identification of these factors, since the coexistence with human suffering and death is perhaps the most stressful factor, as well as the confrontation in making difficult decisions, from which ethical and moral implications are frequently derived, generating occupational stress as physical, mental and emotional wear and tear.

In this regard chapter nine: Roles of the nursing expert in health care malpractice focuses on the background of forensic medicine, the regulatory framework of health care malpractice, and the role of the nursing expert.

Finally, there is chapter ten: International occupational health and safety organizations. In which information is compiled on the current initiatives of each regulatory body for occupational health. These initiatives serve as a basis for reducing health risks, enabling occupational and environmental safety, as well as improving occupational health practices.

The coordinators of the book express our gratitude to the collaborators of this work, guaranteeing the value of the information provided.

We hope that this issue will be to the readers' liking, convinced that the contents of the chapters provide elements for consultation to improve practice in the field of occupational health.

CONTENT

INTRODUCTION 1

CHAPTER 1 4

CHAPTER 2 11

CHAPTER 3 21

CHAPTER 4 30

CHAPTER 5 38

CHAPTER 6 47

CHAPTER 7 56

CHAPTER 8 63

CHAPTER 9 72

CHAPTER 10 83

CHAPTER 1

OCCUPATIONAL HEALTH PROTECTION, PROMOTION AND PREVENTION

Janet Carolina Negrón Espadas** Niusette Asunción Ceballos Avila* Luis Ángel Suaste Sosa* Luis Ángel Suaste Sosa* Luis Ángel Suaste Sosa* Luis Ángel Suaste Sosa* Luis Ángel Suaste Sosa* Luis Ángel Suaste Sosa

"Health Promotion constitutes a global political and social process that encompasses actions aimed at modifying social, labor and economic conditions for a positive impact on individual and collective health."

Ottawa Charter (WHO).

Introduction

The Health Promotion approach has a particular way of contributing: it starts from the dissimilar needs of the population, builds on their capacities and strengths, is collaborative, is intersectoral, is context sensitive and works at various levels: communities, populations, organizations, and institutions working together to establish conditions and environments that ensure health and wellbeing for all people, leaving no one behind. In this context, this chapter will focus on occupational health, with a perspective on its protection, promotion and prevention. One of the main reasons that the impact of occupational health has been affected in recent years is that most working people spend a third of their time in their work area, hence the importance of providing workers with good working conditions, risk protection, personal development and social status.In October 1986, WHO and the Canadian Public Health Association and Health and Welfare Canada organized what would become the first international conference on health promotion, known today as the Ottawa Charter,*Student of the Bachelor's Degree in Nursing. Autonomous University of Yucatan recognizes that the workplace is one of the most important key components of successful health promotion. It states that "The way in which society organizes work should contribute to creating a healthy society. Health promotion generates safe, stimulating, satisfying and enjoyable living and working conditions." With this it is understood that health promotion goes beyond health care and that politics must be involved in making action plans for companies and the care of their workers. [1]

The charter covered five areas of action for health promotion: creating enabling environments, developing a healthy public policy, strengthening the community, developing personal skills, and reorienting health services.

Other conferences were held which gave weight to the development of health promotion in the workplace, such as the III World Conference on Health Promotion held in 1988 in Adelaide, Australia, which recognized the workplace as an environment for the application of health promotion.

The conference in Sundsyvall, Sweden in 1991 addressed the issue of creating health-promoting environments. In 1997, the member countries of the European Network for Workplace Health Promotion adopted the Luxembourg Declaration in which they defined priorities for future activities such as: raising awareness and commitment of company employees to workplace health promotion, developing guidelines for effective practice, identifying and disseminating successful projects, and addressing specific problems resulting from collaboration with small and medium-sized enterprises (SMEs).[1]

Unfortunately, unsafe working conditions are not only found in factories or industrial plants, since any job can have an unfavorable health environment for the worker. The importance of health in the worker will always determine to a large extent the productivity and vitality of this in the workplace, without leaving aside the personal issue. For this reason, health professionals have a fundamental role in the protection and promotion of occupational health of all active personnel during their working time, in addition to this in many companies are hired graduates in nursing who are responsible for providing their services regarding the occupational health of companies, therefore, Therefore, it is important to prepare these professionals so that they can help to carry out strategies for an improvement in occupational health, since they would improve and cause a reduction in the number of occupational accidents, but above all, it would make the personnel of companies more aware of the occupational risks that in some way intervene in their state of health.

Prioritization of the concept of protection, prevention and health promotion in the workplace.

For the development of this interesting topic, it should be mentioned that occupational health is part of a great approach, since workers are important people for the organization or company where they work regardless of the position or area in which they work.Therefore, it is necessary to promote the health, well-being and quality of life of workers, so employers should set goals with respect to occupational health.Likewise, one of the great challenges of public health involves implementing strategies, programs and initiatives in occupational health based mainly on health promotion, prevention and protection.Within the framework of the above considerations, it is necessary to define occupational health, according to the WHO it is "a multidisciplinary activity that promotes and protects the health of workers. This discipline seeks to control accidents and diseases by reducing risk conditions". In other words, it is the reduction or elimination of these factors, of illnesses or accidents in the work area, more precisely in the tasks performed by the worker.[2]

The protection of workers' health implies avoiding exploitation, the risk of contracting diseases, accidents, remuneration for their work, and the risk of being paid for the work they do. The right working conditions are not only conducive to social protection, but also promote personal development opportunities and protect workers against physical and psychosocial risks. Adequate working conditions are not only conducive to social protection, but also favor opportunities for personal development and protect workers against physical and psychosocial risks, as well as having positive effects on health and well-being.[3] It is worth mentioning that occupational safety and health are two closely related activities, aimed at ensuring working conditions capable of maintaining the level of health of workers.The term health promotion implies providing information and skills to workers and promoting improvements in environmental conditions.The definition is constantly being modified in accordance with the current regulations. [4]

Therefore, health promotion implies that individuals use their skills, resources and knowledge to satisfy their basic needs and advocate for the respect of their rights, justice, peace, as well as the satisfaction of their basic needs for housing, food and clothing. The health of working people is directly connected to the productivity of the company.Likewise, prevention seeks to promote the improvement of occupational health and safety, through the application of measures and the development of activities necessary to avoid or reduce the risks derived from working conditions, considering risk assessment as a fundamental tool. This must be one of the fundamental pillars in the organization and management of any company, insofar as it has human capital that must be cared for and protected to ensure the proper functioning of the company, as well as the health and quality of the work performed by this human team.[5]

Thus, the practice of occupational health nursing is derived from a synthesis of knowledge obtained basically from medicine, public health, social sciences and theories of management and labor law. Occupational nursing has as its main objective The objective is to contribute to the physical and mental well-being of workers in their work area.

Among the functions of occupational nursing are:
• To protect workers from health risks, maintaining a healthy environment for workers to perform their work without compromising their health.
• To know the employees in a psychological way.

• Promote organizational systems that foster a positive environment, promote safety and eliminate risks.

In relation to the above, it is important to articulate the actions of protection, prevention and promotion of health to the official Mexican standards, the Federal Labor Law and the Political Constitution of the United Mexican States, since these legislations help to regulate the protection of labor rights of all Mexicans. All of the above, to contribute to the health and psychological well-being of workers.

Lines of action for health promotion in the workplace.

From the public health point of view, there are different lines of action that help and give great impact and credibility to health promotion, regarding occupational health. These form an important part of occupational health, since they can be used to create initiatives, programs and public policies. The lines of action for the promotion of occupational health are: [6,7,8]

1. Development of healthy public policies and legislation.
2. Creation and protection of healthy environments.
3. Strengthening of individual and collective potentialities.

With respect to line of action I. **Elaboration of healthy public policies and legislation,** for the promotion of good public policies in occupational health, there are different agencies and different sectors responsible for defining policies. related to the determinants of occupational health. The means to be used to make this line of action effective are varied, including fiscal measures, legislation, organizational changes, among others.

Leading organizations include:

First of all, the International Labor Organization (ILO) develops and applies a culture of safety and preventive health in the workplace. In 2003, the ILO instituted April 28 as World Day for Safety and Health at Work, to highlight the need to prevent occupational diseases and accidents, using social dialogue as a support point. [9]

Secondly, the Pan American Health Organization (PAHO) considers the workplace to be a priority environment for health promotion in the 21st century; it states that occupational health and healthy work environments are people's most precious assets.There are regulations regarding the promotion, protection and prevention of occupational health in the United Mexican States. Mexico has a political constitution of the United Mexican States, the federal safety regulations, the federal labor and occupational health law, and other systems that are applicable in the country regarding occupational safety and health, such as the Mexican Official Standards (NOM).The Political Constitution of the United States of Mexico is the supreme law that governs our country since it contains precepts related to the safety and health of workers, the most important points it covers are: [10]

• Everyone has the right to health protection.
• Every company shall be obliged to provide its workers with on-the-job training.

• Employers shall be responsible for accidents at work and for workers' illnesses suffered in the course of their work, therefore the company shall pay compensation according to the consequences that affect the worker, such as death or disability. temporary/permanent. This liability will exist even if the employer contracts the work through an intermediary.

• In specific labor matters, the regulation is the Federal Labor Law of 1970, in which the obligation is for the employer to provide and guarantee the safety and health of the workers. The ninth title mentions about the regulation of occupational hazards that occur in work areas aimed at protecting the safety and health of salaried workers in Mexico.

• In the area of occupational safety and health the standard is the Federal Regulation on Occupational Safety and Health of 2014, this law replaces the past Federal Regulation on Occupational Safety, Hygiene and Environment. It establishes to incorporate more concrete obligations regarding the prevention and management of certain specific risks in workplaces and workplaces.

• Development of the employer's responsibilities in relation to occupational health and safety protection, there is a series of specific regulations governing the prevention and management of specific risks, as well as organizational aspects.

Regarding line of action II. **Creation and protection of healthy environments,** the person and the work environment have a very close relationship, where the worker performs his corresponding activities, for that reason, healthy work areas must be provided so that the well-being of the worker is very good and with the least number of occupational risks, that is to say, the modifications in the environment in which people usually develop (at work or in their recreation) affect positively or negatively in a significant way their health situation.

Unfortunately, workers do not have healthy environments in their work area, which triggers various accidents and risks to the health of workers. To avoid this, the Political Constitution of the United Mexican States refers to the following:

"The employer shall be obliged to observe, in accordance with the nature of his business, the legal precepts on hygiene and safety in the premises of his The company is obliged to adopt adequate measures to prevent accidents in the use of machines, instruments and work materials, as well as to organize it in such a way as to guarantee the health and life of the workers, as well as of pregnant women and their unborn children. The laws shall contain, to this effect, the appropriate sanctions in each case."

On the other hand, line of action III. **Strengthening of individual and collective potentialities,** contemplates information, health education and the modification of diverse attitudes to maintain or remain in a healthy work environment, with the purpose of a good social and personal development.

This line of action is a fundamental part of health promotion and prevention, as it refers to the phrase "education begins at home", since knowing, reflecting, teaching and asserting our rights as workers helps us to have very good job opportunities with the least amount of risks to our health.

That is why one of the most propitious ways to enforce this line of action is through the development of educational processes in companies focused on stimulating the individual skills of workers in daily life, decision making and problem solving.

This line of action is closely linked to line of action II, because everyone can demand their labor rights for the creation of a good working environment according to the needs that arise at work, for example, demand good lighting and ventilation in the work area and even change old electronic devices that somehow put the worker's health at risk.

Conclusions

A key starting point is to recognize that the worker has a great impact on the development and process in the different work areas in which he/she works. However, not enough measures are taken for a work environment that allows the development of their skills without the exposure to different health risks to which they are subjected. It is currently known that the importance of public policies and all legislation in the place where employment is exercised is undeniable, since they provide a support for of all activities carried out during working hours. However, there is a deficiency of these and a vague knowledge of these laws that protect workers. Teaching companies about the promotion of occupational health, as well as its prevention and protection, will help to have a large number of workers who know their rights and strengthen their cognitive skills about the risks and protection of their health in the work environment where they work. When analyzing the three lines of action focused on occupational health and the basic tools of Health Promotion, we find the ideal field to develop the postulates of this chapter, the methods and techniques of intervention that could be applied from the individual to the collective. Knowing these lines of action provides the knowledge, abilities, skills, coordination, social mobilization for the ethical formation that privileges the human being as an integral and collective being in a labor field. This chapter reflects on the ideal conditions for professionals to recreate their profession in an interdisciplinary, inter-sectorial and inter-organizational environment, with the usual difficulties inherent to this type of experiences and spaces. But also in an environment that favors the positive, physical, emotional and social health. It is important that companies take into consideration the health of their workers, which in turn leads to lower absenteeism, higher motivation, higher productivity, lower turnover, a positive image and a solid corporate social responsibility. The presence of occupational health in a company is of vital importance, since in addition to ensuring the highest physical, mental and social well-being of employees, it seeks to establish and sustain a safe and healthy work environment. If an institution is not governed by occupational health standards, it will be prone to enter into external legal disputes by the workers who have been affected, and therefore this will have an impact on its productivity and permanence in the market.

Referrals

1. ILO. Occupational health promotion and well-being at work.[Internet]2015 (cited 24 June 2022). Available from: https://www.ilo.org/global/topics/safety-and-health-at-work/areasofwork/workplace-health-promotion-and-well-being/lang--en/index.htm.
2. University of Nariño. Occupational health. [Internet]2012 (cited June 26, 2022). Available from: http://www.scielo.org.co/pdf/reus/v14n1/v14n1a08.pdf
3. Blanco Gomez, Gisela, Workers' health, [Internet]2016 (cited June 10, 2022). Available from: https://www.redalyc.org/pdf/3758/375851163008.pdf
4. Government of Spain. Salud Laboral. [Internet]2015 (cited June 10, 2022). Available from: https://saludlaboralydiscapacidad.org/salud-laboral/que-es/
5. WHO. Workers' health protection. [Internet]2017 (cited June 10, 2022). Available from: https://www.who.int/es/news-room/fact- sheets/detail/protecting-workers'-health#:~:text=The%20good%20conditions%20of%20work,effects%20positive%20for%20health.
6. PAHO. Health Promotion. [Internet]2015 (cited June 10, 2022). Available from: https://www.paho.org/es/temas/promocion-salud
7. Government of Spain. Salud Laboral. [Internet]2015 (cited June 11, 2022).Disponiblen: https://istas.net/salud-laboral
8. National University of Colombia.Workplace health promotion. [Internet]2015 (cited June 24, 2022). Available from: https://scielo.isciii.es/pdf/mesetra/v56n220/original2.pdf
9. Garrosa Hernández Eva, Carmona Cobo Isabel. Occupational health and well-being: Incorporation of positive models to the understanding and prevention of psychosocial risks at work. Med. segur. trab. [Internet]. 2011 [cited 2022 Jun 24] ; 57(Suppl 1): 224-238. Available from: http://scielo.isciii.es/scielo.php?script=sci_arttext&pid=S0465-546X2011000500014&lng=en.
10. DOF. Political Constitution of the United Mexican States. [Internet]2021 (cited June 24, 2022). Available at: https://www.diputados.gob.mx/LeyesBiblio/pdf/CPEUM.pdf

CHAPTER 2

EVALUATION AND DIAGNOSIS OF WORKERS' HEALTH.

Janet Carolina Negrón Espadas** Paola Alessandra Alonzo Aguilar* Regina Mercedes Qui Varguez* Regina Mercedes Qui Varguez* Regina Mercedes Qui Varguez* Regina Mercedes Qui Varguez

"If you don't pursue what you want, you will never get it. If you don't ask, the answer will always be no. If you don't ask, the answer will always be no. If you don't step forward, you will always be in the same place."

Nora Roberts.

Introduction

Work is one of the fundamental pillars of society that dignifies and empowers the person who performs it; it can be defined as any manual or intellectual labor that is performed in order to obtain a remunerative salary.[1]

Worldwide, almost 800,000 deaths occur annually as a result of occupational injuries and 11,000,000 to occupational diseases; in Latin America and the Caribbean, 300 workers die daily due to occupational accidents, which is why, in Mexico, the federal labor law establishes that a decent job must ensure and respect the integrity of the worker, which is achieved by generating an environment with adequate occupational health.[2,3] Occupational health promotes and protects the health of workers, and is defined as the state of highest and optimal well-being of a worker in the main spheres: physical, mental and social, including the promotion, maintenance and prevention of the worker's health in the workplace.[4]

*Student of the Bachelor's Degree in Nursing. Autonomous University of Yucatan

**Career Professor. Faculty of Nursing. Autonomous University of Yucatan

In the workplace, there are countless risk factors that expose workers and make them susceptible to damage or repercussions, including physical, chemical and mechanical factors, among others, which are considered relevant to carry out an evaluation and integrate these diagnoses in terms of occupational health in different companies, since from this diagnosis derive the different programs and interventions for the well-being of workers.[5]

In this chapter the most important points to be taken into account at the time of carrying out health evaluations and diagnoses of workers, the importance of this topic is justified in the current regulations and in the fact that maintaining a comprehensive welfare in the worker raises their labor competence and productivity, which in turn improves the working environment, the quality of life of the person and finally represents a fact that favors the economy of society and the country.

Occupational risk factors

Work is an important pillar for society, since it is an activity that generates the growth of a country and its inhabitants. Therefore, it is important to highlight the importance of the worker's health, since health conditions the development, competence and productivity of the employee.Therefore, companies and governments are aware of the various regulations that support the fundamental right to safe work, however, occupational accidents continue to occur frequently around the world, because of this it is necessary to create safety policies for the prevention of occupational hazards, however, However, before creating these policies and legislation, it is essential to recognize the risk factors to which a worker is exposed at the time of performing his role as an employee, since knowing the risk factors facilitates the identification of the hazards to which the employee is exposed and this expedites the prevention of occupational accidents.[6]

Occupational risk factors or occupational hazards are unforeseen events or conditions that can endanger the integrity of the worker, these come from the environment or surroundings, from the equipment or machinery used and even from the operator himself, due to which the following classification is made[7]:

Physical risk factors: these are those related to or conditioned by the physical environment and include the different types of energies present in the environment that can harm the worker's integrity or have the potential to cause harm. In turn, they can be subclassified as follows[5,8]:

- Mechanical energy: noise and vibrations.
- Electromagnetic energy: ionizing and non-ionizing radiations
- Calorific energy: heat or cold.

Chemical risk factor: any chemical substance of organic and inorganic nature, natural or synthetic, whose exposure by inhalation, ingestion or skin contact may cause corrosive, toxic, irritant or asphyxiating effects that endanger the employee's health. They are further subclassified into[5,7]:

- According to their physical state: solids, liquids, gases, dusts, chemical fumes, mists, vapors, aerosols, fumes, fibers, sprays,
- According to their chemical effects: irritants, asphyxiants, anesthetics and narcotics, toxics, carcinogens, teratogens and mutagens, caustics and corrosives, sensitizers.

Biological risk factor: refers to the high probability of exposure to microorganisms that can trigger a deviation in human health, including viruses, bacteria, fungi, parasites that are pathogenic in nature and are acquired due to the work activity performed.[9]

Psychosocial risk factors: The Mexican Official Standard NOM-035-STPS-2018, Psychosocial risk factors at work-Identification, analysis and prevention defines the psychosocial risk factor as "those that can cause anxiety disorders, non-organic sleep-wake cycle and severe stress and adaptation, derived from the nature of the job functions, the type of workday and exposure to severe traumatic events or acts of workplace violence to the worker, by the work developed. They include hazardous and unsafe conditions in the work environment; workloads when they exceed the worker's capacity. of the worker; lack of control over the work (possibility of influencing the organization and development of the work when the process allows it); work shifts longer than those foreseen in the Federal Labor Law, shift rotation that includes night shifts and night shifts without recovery and rest periods; interference in the work-family relationship, and negative leadership and negative relationships at work "[10].

Ergonomic risk factors: are defined in the Mexican Official Standard NOM- 036-1-STPS-2018, Ergonomic Risk Factors at Work-Identification, analysis, prevention and control. Part 1: Manual handling of loads, as "those that can lead to over physical effort, repetitive movements or forced postures in the work performed, with the consequent fatigue, errors, accidents and occupational diseases, derived from the design of the facilities, machinery, equipment, tools or work station.[11]

Mechanical risk factor: This type of risk refers to those factors that exert a spontaneous or mechanical action of tools, machines, equipment, which can cause injuries to workers who use these types of mechanisms. Examples in this group include trapping, falling objects, collisions with objects, blows and cuts from tools. [12]

Electrical risk factor: This is constituted by the possibility of the electric current coming into contact with the human body, which can occur as a direct contact (by touching an active live part) or by indirect contact such as that produced by touching an element or mass accidentally put under voltage.[13]

Locational risk factor: This refers to those conditions in the facilities or work areas that can cause accidents if they are not kept in adequate conditions; this risk is one of the most common and important in occupational accidents, since it involves deficiencies such as lack of cleanliness, lack of signage and poor condition of the facilities or elements with which workers come into contact.[14]

Physical-chemical risk factor: This type of risk includes chemical substances, materials and objects that can be a source of danger for the worker, such as fires or explosions derived from the incorrect handling of the aforementioned aspects.[15]

Diagnosis of worker's health

As mentioned above, it is important for nursing professionals to monitor the health status of workers, from the moment the worker applies to join a company until he/she is hired, for which tools are used to determine the general state of health. This diagnosis should be carried out under a holistic approach to the individual, and the occupational risks to which he or she is exposed due to the job or working conditions should be identified, as well as the reasons for prolonged absenteeism.[16,17]

With regard to pregnant women who are at work, it is relevant that they can validate the right to the issuance of the certificate of maternity disability, which is extended for 84 days, It is important that the woman notifies her pregnancy as soon as possible so that a reevaluation of the risk factors to which she is exposed and which may cause some inconvenience in this vulnerable stage of pregnancy can be made. It is important to mention that this occupational health diagnosis should not be limited to the gestation process, but also includes the breastfeeding stage, so it is essential to enforce the right described above. Likewise, pregnant women shall not perform work that requires lifting, pulling or pushing heavy weights, or work that causes trepidation or standing for long periods of time. [16]

Obviously, qualified health professionals will be in charge of performing the medical studies necessary for the diagnosis of the worker's current health. The diagnostic tools include clinical history, physical examination, complementary tests such as laboratories (blood biometry, blood group and Rh factor, urine test), specific complementary tests according to the type of risk and exposure (musculoskeletal assessment, chest X-ray, spirometry, audiometry) and toxicological tests, which include tests based on urine tests, blood tests and exhaled air analysis. [17]

In addition, according to the results obtained, the worker's aptitudes to adapt to the conditions of the job position will be determined. In other words, the findings The clinical tests will allow the identification of diseases or pre-pathological conditions to take the necessary precautions to perform their work. In this way, a worker will be declared unfit if he/she presents sequelae of pathologies or accidents that limit him/her and make his/her performance and work impossible. In this sense, the health diagnosis is considered a labor right for employees and an obligation for employers.[17]

In a complementary manner, the Federal Labor Law, in Title Five Bis, Article 174 establishes that "those over fifteen and under eighteen years of age must obtain a medical certificate attesting to their aptitude for work and submit to the medical examinations periodically ordered by the corresponding labor authorities. Without these requirements, no employer may use their services.[3]

Therefore, in order to deepen on the diagnosis of safety and health at work, the Mexican Official Standard NOM-030-STPS-2009, Preventive services of safety and health at work - Functions and activities, talks about the comprehensive diagnosis of hazardous and unsafe conditions in terms of equipment used for the performance of work, as well as physical, chemical and biological agents that represent a risk factor for the worker, therefore, it is important to emphasize these regulatory requirements to have adequate safety and health in the workplace; It is also important to mention the corrective and preventive actions that are part of this occupational health care and that are so essential to take responsibility in these aspects and in emergency care.[18]

Occupational risk assessment

Risk assessment is a systematic process carried out with the purpose of identifying and estimating the magnitude of risk factors, conditions and practices present in a work environment, in order to gather the information and data necessary for the employer and the company to generate preventive measures and create a culture of safety and accident prevention. This process consists of 3 main phases: risk identification, risk analysis and risk assessment:[19]

1. **Risk identification.** The purpose of this phase is to determine and specify the risks and uncertainties that endanger the worker during the performance of his work. In this section it is important to describe in a timely manner those places and circumstances that have the potential to cause injury or harm to the employee, for this it is vital that the collection of data from all places within the company and places related to this that have these abnormal circumstances that put at risk the welfare of people is performed, To facilitate this section, a previously established basic list of possible hazards can be used, such as the one shown in Table 1, or alternatively, one can be projected whose specificity is more related to the activity or branch of the company.[19,20]

Table 1. Risks in the workplace.

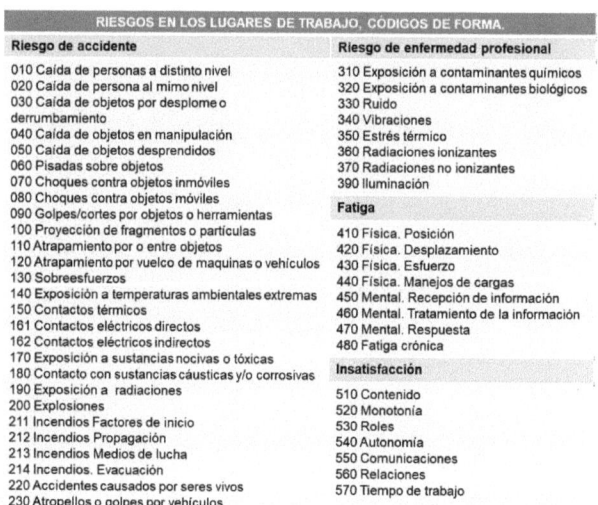

2. **Risk analysis.** In this phase, the objective is to understand and encompass the characteristics of the risks, as well as the probabilities and different scenarios, since it is important to understand that a single risk can be multi-causal and can have a variety of consequences, therefore, this risk analysis must have reliable techniques, taking into account different results to make the most timely and corrective decisions for improvement, since the magnitude of the risk must also be analyzed, as well as

taking into account the nature of the events, the probability of occurrence, the interaction of factors and levels of sensitivity and confidence of instruments and analysis techniques to develop strategies and treatments to prevent such risks.[19]

3. **Risk assessment.** The purpose of this last phase is to assist in decision making, since it involves determining the results of the risk analysis and knowing when additional action is required in order to have an adequate assessment, since it is possible to choose not to take further action, to consider additional options and analyses for risk treatment, as well as to continue with existing controls and measures or to restate objectives, all of this for the improvement and effectiveness in the treatment and control of occupational risk.[19]

Table 2 shows how, by crossing the variables of probability and consequence, the final risk assessment is obtained, which can be considered trivial, tolerable, moderate, important and intolerable. Table 3 specifies the measures to be followed in the treatment of risks depending on the analysis and assessment and the results obtained.

Evaluation method to determine the magnitude of the risk

		CONSECUENCIA		
		Ligeramente dañino	Dañino	Extremadamente dañino
PROBABILIDAD	Baja	Riesgo trivial (T)	Riesgo tolerable (To)	Riesgo moderado (M)
	Media	Riesgo tolerable (To)	Riesgo moderado (M)	Riesgo importante (I)
	Alta	Riesgo moderado (M)	Riesgo importante (I)	Riesgo intolerable (IN)

Table 3. Corrective and preventive measures

Riesgo	Acción y temporización
Trivial (T)	No se requiere una acción específica.
Tolerable (TO)	No se necesita mejorar la acción preventiva. Sin embargo, se deben considerar soluciones más rentables o mejoras que no supongan una carga económica importante. Se requieren comprobaciones periódicas para asegurar que se mantiene la eficacia de las medidas de control.
Moderado (M)	Se deben hacer esfuerzos para reducir el riesgo, determinando las inversiones precisas. Las medidas para reducir el riesgo deben implantarse en un período determinado. Cuando el riesgo moderado está asociado con consecuencias extremadamente dañinas, se precisará una acción posterior para establecer, con más precisión, la probabilidad de daño como base para determinar la necesidad de mejora de las medidas de control.
Importante (I)	No debe comenzarse el trabajo hasta que se haya reducido el riesgo. Puede que se precisen recursos considerables para controlar el riesgo. Cuando el riesgo corresponda a un trabajo que se está realizando, debe remediarse el problema en un tiempo inferior al de los riesgos moderados.
Intolerable (IN)	El trabajo no debe comenzar ni continuar hasta que se reduzca el riesgo. Si no es posible reducir el riesgo, incluso con recursos ilimitados, debe prohibirse el trabajo.

In this regard, the Ministry of Labor and Social Welfare (STPS), in the area of occupational safety and health, establishes the regulations for the evaluation of risk factors in the following Official Mexican Standards21:

- NOM-001-STPS-2008 Buildings, premises, facilities and areas in workplaces. - Safety conditions

- NOM-002-STPS-2010 Prevention and protection against fire in workplaces. - Safety conditions

- NOM-004-STPS-1999. Protection systems and safety devices in machinery and equipment used in the workplace.

- NOM-005-STPS1998 Handling, transport and storage of hazardous chemicals.

- NOM-006-STPS-2014 Handling and storage of materials - Occupational safety and health conditions.

- NOM-009-STPS-2011 Safety conditions for working at heights
- NOM-020-STPS-2011 Pressure vessels, cryogenic vessels and steam generators or boilers Operation. - Safety conditions

- NOM-022-STPS2008 Static electricity in workplaces. - Safety conditions

- NOM-027-STPS2008. Welding and cutting activities. - Safety and hygiene conditions

- NOM-029-STPS-2011 Maintenance of electrical installations in workplaces. Safety conditions

- NOM-035-STPS-2018 Psychosocial risk factors at work-Identification, analysis and prevention.

- NOM-036-1-STPS-2018 Ergonomic risk factors at work- identification, analysis, prevention and control.

- NOM 010-STPS-1999. Handling, transport, processing and storage of chemical substances capable of generating contamination in the work environment. - Safety and hygiene conditions

- NOM-011-STPS2001. Noise in workplaces. - Safety and hygiene conditions

- NOM-012-STPS-2012 Ionizing radiation. - Safety and health conditions in workplaces where ionizing radiation sources are handled.

- NOM-013-STPS-1993 Non-ionizing electromagnetic radiation. - Health and safety conditions in workplaces where they are generated.

- NOM-014-STPS-2000 Occupational exposure to abnormal environmental pressures. - Safety and hygiene conditions

- NOM-015- STPS-2001 Elevated or depressed thermal conditions. - Safety and hygiene conditions

- NOM-024- STPS-2001 Vibrations in workplaces. - Safety and hygiene conditions
- NOM-025-STPS-2008 Lighting conditions in the workplace.

In addition, the Ministry of Labor and Social Welfare (STPS) has a Self-Management Program for Occupational Safety and Health in which a "Guide for the Evaluation of Compliance with Occupational Safety and Health Regulations" is developed, which establishes an instrument to evaluate those regulations in order to adopt measures in favor of occupational safety and health.[22]

Conclusions

It is important to mention the relevance and impact that this topic confers, since it has been seen and proven the different risks and problems that arise in the workplace, and derived from this the damage that can be caused to workers, which is why the diagnosis and evaluation of occupational health should be an intrinsic and fundamental issue for companies, as this can achieve great progress in terms of safety and protection of workers.Learning about occupational risk factors, the different types of diagnostics that should be carried out with workers and the process for assessing occupational risk suggest a new outlook for creating safe, dignified and compliant work environments and monitoring regulations. By promoting the implementation of a culture of safety and prevention in the work environment of the various companies and jobs, it favors the reduction and reduction of occupational risks and accidents, this in turn implies that there is a continuous growth in the company, as it maintains and increases the welfare of the worker, which benefits in the fact that production and labor effectiveness are increased, thus helping the economy and development of the community.

References

1. Romero, M. Meaning of work from the psychology of work. A historical, psychological and social review. Psychology from the Caribbean. Universidad del Norte. [Internet] 2017. [Cited June 10, 2022] 34(2):120-138. Disponible en: http://www.scielo.org.co/pdf/psdc/v34n2/2011-7485-psdc-34-02-00120.pdf
2. Pan American Health Organization. Workers' Health: Resources - Frequently Asked Questions. [Internet]. [Cited June 10, 2022] Available from: https://www3.paho.org/hq/index.php?option=com_content&view=article&id=1527:workers-health-resources&Itemid=1349&limitstart=2&lang=en.
3. Official Gazette of the Federation. Federal Labor Law. [Internet]. 2015 [Cited June 10, 2022]. Available at: https://www.diputados.gob.mx/LeyesBiblio/pdf/LFT.pdf
4. State Foundation for the Prevention of Occupational Risks. Salud Laboral [Internet]. [Cited June 12, 2022. Available at: https://saludlaboralydiscapacidad.org/salud-laboral/que-es/
5. Henao F. Integral diagnosis of working conditions and health. 2nd ed. Bogotá. Ecoe Ediciones; 2012.
6. HISCOX Spain. Safety at work: occupational risk factors. [Internet]. 2018. [Cited June 12, 2022] Available from: https://www.hiscox.es/factores-de-riesgo-laboral.
7. Catholic University of San Pablo. Know what is a risk factor in occupational health. [Internet] [Cited June 12, 2022] Available at: https://postgrado.ucsp.edu.pe/articulos/factor-riesgo-salud-ocupacional/
8. Mining Safety. Physical risk factors at work. [Internet]. 2018. [Cited June 12, 2022] Available from: https://www.revistaseguridadminera.com/operaciones-mineras/factores-de- riesgo-fisico-en-el-trabajo/.
9. Vera, R., Navas, Y., Guales, I. Main occupational risk factors affecting health care workers. Rev. Sci. Sci. [Internet]. 2017. [Cited June 15, 2022]. 3(2), 106-130. Available from: https://dialnet.unirioja.es/descarga/articulo/5889728.pdf
10. Official Journal of the Federation. NORMA Oficial Mexicana NOM-035-STPS-2018, Factores de riesgo psicosocial en el trabajo-Identificación, análisis y prevención. [Cited June 15, 2022]. Available at: https://www.dof.gob.mx/nota_detalle.php?codigo=5541828&fecha=23/10/2018#gsc.tab=0
11. Official Journal of the Federation. NORMA Oficial Mexicana NOM-036-1-STPS-2018, Factores de riesgo ergonómico en el Trabajo-Identificación, análisis, prevención y control. Part 1: Manual handling of loads. [Cited June 15, 2022]. Available at: https://www.dof.gob.mx/normasOficiales/7468/stps11_C/stps11_C.html
12. Martínez S. Identification and evaluation of mechanical and ergonomic risks in the personnel of the distribution company Víctor Mocoso e Hijos de la Ciudad de Cuenca. Ecuador. Salesian Polytechnic University; 2015.
13. Portal of Occupational Risks of Teaching Workers. Foundation for the prevention of occupational hazards. [Internet]. 2015. [Cited 14 June 2022]. Available at: https://riesgoslaborales.saludlaboral.org/portal- preventivo/ riesgos-laborales/ riesgos-relacionados-con-la-seguridad-con-la-seguridad-en-el-el- trabajo/electricidad/.
14. Carlosama J., Mejía M., Bonilla A., Córdoba M. DETERMINATION OF THE

LOCATIVE RISK FACTORS THAT DIMINISH THE LABOR PERFORMANCE OF THE WORKERS OF THE JUGOS LA JARRA COMPANY. [Internet]. 2019. [Cited June 14, 2022]. Available from: https://repository.ean.edu.co/bitstream/handle/10882/9754/BonillaAura2019?sequence=1&isAllowed=y.

15. Technological Institute of Culiacan. Physical risk factors. [Internet]. 2017. [Cited June 14, 2022]. Available at: SIG-IN-F-P-P-35-07-Table-of-Physical-Risk-Factors-OK-1.docx (live.com).

16. Rodríguez M. WORKERS' HEALTH SURVEILLANCE IN THE CONTEXT OF OCCUPATIONAL HAZARD PREVENTION. QUALITY AND PREVENTIVE USEFULNESS OF HEALTH EXAMINATIONS. [Internet]. 2017. [Cited 12 June 2022]. Available at: http://hdl.handle.net/10803/396181

17. University of Guanajuato. Company health diagnosis. [Internet]. 2018. [Cited 12 June 2022]. Available from: https://blogs.ugto.mx/enfermeriaenlinea/unidad-didactica-4-diagnostico-de-salud- de-la-empresa/.

18. Official Journal of the Federation. NORMA Oficial Mexicana NOM-030-STPS-2009, Servicios preventivos de seguridad y salud en el trabajo-Funciones y actividades. [Internet]. 2009. [Cited June 14, 2022]. Disponible en: https://www.dof.gob.mx/normasOficiales/3923/stps/stps.htm%23:~:text%3DNORMA%2520Oficial%2520Mexicana%2520NOM%252D030%2Cel%2520trabajo%252DFunciones%2520y%2520actividades%26text%3DEstablecer%2520las%2520funciones%2520y%2520actividades%2Caccidentes%2520y%2.

19. ISO. Risk Management-Guidelines. [Internet]. 2018. [Cited June 1, 2022]. Available from: https://www.iso.org/obp/ui#iso:std:iso:31000:ed-2:v1:es

20. Mutua Universal. Occupational risk prevention for SMEs: Risk assessment. 2017. [Cited June 15, 2022]. Available at: https://www.mutuauniversal.net/flippingbooks/16/data/downloads/16_eval_riesgo s.pdf.

21. Mexican Institute of Social Security. Occupational Health Surveillance. [Internet]. 2020. [Cited June 15, 2022]. Available at: https://elssa.imss.gob.mx/files/3.3.19_Evaluacion_medio_amb.pdf

22. Ministry of Labor and Social Welfare. Self-management Program in Occupational Safety and Health. [Internet]. 2015. [Cited June 15, 2022]. Available at: https://autogestionsst.stps.gob.mx/Proyecto/Content/doctos/Gu%C3%ADaECNSST.pdf.

CHAPTER 3

DETECTION OF RISKS AND WORKING CONDITIONS

Aurora Sierra Canto ** Aurora Sierra Canto
Karla América Fuentes Elizarraraz * Jesús Elías Martínez Torres * Jesús Elías Martínez Torres * Karla América Fuentes Elizarraraz * Jesús Elías Martínez Torres
Free jobs are those in which the rights of the employee are respected and where the laws are therefore fair.

Maximilien Robespierre.

Introduction

If we go back a few hundred years, we have that, in prehistoric times, the concern for identifying risks did not exist, although it is still true that man was always characterized by trying to protect himself from the dangers that threatened him. If we take prehistoric man as a reference, then it is identifiable that he did not notice the risk as something potential that could affect him, that man dressed in a rudimentary way was concerned about the danger that was visually noticeable, giving some examples: A rushing river, a large and ferocious animal, a strong storm, etc. And as everything is part of a constant evolution, he most likely understood that the above was a danger, because at some point he must have been a spectator of how a man drowned in a river or an animal killed his fellow man.The history of the human species is related to a continuous exposure to adversity and its initial concern was always the demand for security and the cancellation of the risks that threatened its extinction and, speaking of something more complex, man as we know him today exists thanks to the success of his ancestors in facing dangers. [1]

*Student of the Bachelor's Degree in Nursing. Autonomous University of Yucatan

**Career Professor. Faculty of Nursing. Autonomous University of Yucatan

Occupational risk is defined as those hazards that may exist in a specific profession or work area, susceptible to cause accidents that may cause some damage or health problem, both physical and psychological. [2]

Risk detection in the workplace includes a range of activities involving individuals and communities, all aimed at preventing occupational hazards, the main objective of which is to identify health problems and thus seek preventive interventions. [3]

In the ILO's constitution it is possible to read the following fragment: "Whereas conditions of labor exist involving such injustice, hardship and privation to large numbers of people as to constitute a menace to universal peace and harmony; and whereas the improvement of these conditions is urgently required (...)". All of the above emphasizes the importance of establishing humane working conditions to build sustainable and peaceful societies. Working conditions are a rather broad area, in which working hours (working time and rest periods), financial remuneration, physical condition and the demands made on employees must be taken into consideration. To tell the truth, working conditions play a fundamental role in the relationship between employee, employer and company, especially because people want more than just a job where they can earn money, they also have certain aspirations such as fair wages and schedules, with the intention of achieving a balance between work, family and personal life, taking into account that human beings spend almost half of their lives fulfilling the responsibilities of a job.[4]

The risk of the people working in the different facilities must be supervised by the employers in a responsible manner, each worker must work in decent working conditions and it is the job of the health professional to actively participate in the detection of occupational hazards to ensure safe working conditions in all possible areas. For all of the above reasons, this chapter will address the relationship that nursing personnel have in the detection of risks in a work area and the conditions that lead to them.

Legal basis of occupational safety

To properly establish the terms "safety and health at work" it is essential to take into account the safety and health diagnosis within the work area, in order to analyze the potential risks for exposed workers.Likewise, workers and employers must comply with their obligations with respect to the regulations and laws in force, especially those described in the Mexican Official Standard NOM - 030 - STPS - 2009: Preventive Occupational Health and Safety Services - functions and activities. Considering as a frame of reference section 6 of said standard.[5]

Within the framework of the above considerations, a useful tool for the detection of health risks is the safety diagnosis. By way of example, this list can include the personal protective equipment used by the employee, as well as machinery, tools, means of transport, materials and energy sources. Therefore, some references point out that it is essential to evaluate aspects such as the above, especially if you want to avoid employee visits to emergency rooms.In some labor institutions risk agents are used, which are classified as physical, chemical and biological. Each element has properties capable of injuring the worker if the appropriate safety measures are not used. For this reason, the governing body, health and safety committees and health professionals must evaluate the exposure time with workers, considering the potential health risks, either by direct or indirect exposure respectively.On the other hand, it is imperative to assess the risks in the workplace, as they may affect workers when they are performing their activities. According to the applicable laws, it is important to identify and make known the relative and integral risks, for which a specific area within the company will be designated. The above must be based on the number of workers that the company or institution has. On the other hand currently the term "Working Conditions" is not directly mentioned in the 2030 declaration of the Sustainable Development Goals (SDGs), but, it is possible to read aspects related to it in various goals and targets, for example: Target 5.4 of the SDGs specifies the complicated situation of domestic workers and private caregivers; target

8.5 calls for equal pay for work of equal value, target 8.8 speaks of the promotion of safe and secure working environments, target 10.4 calls for the adoption of appropriate wage policies to achieve greater equality, while target 16.6 points to the creation of accountable institutions, which are indispensable for the improvement of working conditions.[4]

Risk detection

Health professionals within the workplace team have the role of identifying and determining the health status of workers. The main activities that can be performed range from clinical evaluations, routine examinations, health monitoring and other activities focused on health surveillance where the skills and knowledge of a nursing professional are required. This is why companies and different organizations should also be concerned about maintaining a close relationship with nursing professionals, with the intention of making ideal interventions with respect to prevalent health problems.[6]

For this reason, the impact and scope of reviews depends on the hazards in the company, the number of workers affected, but also on the history of problems or incidents, including malfunctions.Likewise, the company must determine the elements that will be subject to evaluation, with respect to the facilities, periodic or regulatory reviews will be carried out. These reviews will evaluate ventilation, lighting, signaling, elevators or control and emergency detection facilities, i.e., to generate pertinent occupational diagnoses to prevent harm to workers.[7]

Surveillance and working conditions

The nursing community that works in occupational health should be related to and involved in environmental monitoring in the workplace, so it is convenient to emphasize that the professional has a major role in the creation of supervisory programs with the intention of identifying potential risks to the health of workers.[6]

Some measures to be implemented could be: tours and inspections in the work area, achieving in a synergic way a familiarization of the health personnel with the work site, the processes involved in the production of the company and being able to notify and provide the necessary materials to preserve the safety of workers in each area.[6]

Whenever a risk is identified, effective strategies should be implemented in order to measure exposure levels as well as the potential impact on the operator's health. Accordingly, the nursing professional must have the ability to identify the specific areas of interaction, which are: the environment, the causative agent and the host, of course this function can be developed in combination with other health professionals.

Occupational supervision scenarios

In relation to the subject, the services of nursing personnel have shown a significant increase with a presence in different work areas, among which we can highlight manufacturing in textile factories, companies dedicated to pharmaceuticals, food, furniture and construction materials.Therefore, it is important that the nursing staff identifies that the company has the follow-up of the document entitled "Diagnosis of safety and hygiene at work", which is the basis for all preventive measures to be implemented, because when a company wants to reduce accidents and diseases, the first step is to analyze their activities and know their production processes For this reason, the following is a format that is useful in the verification of existing safety and hygiene conditions in the area.[8]

Table 1. Occupational health and safety checklist.

Table 1. Checklist of Safety and Hygiene conditions of the Existing work			
Safety and hygiene element of the work	Yes apply	No apply	Regulations
Steam generators and vessels pressurized			NOM-020-STPS-2002
2. Protection and protection devices safety in machinery, equipment and accessories.			NOM-004-STPS-1999
Welding and cutting activities			NOM-027-STPS-2000
3. Environmental conditions			
Noise			NOM-011-STPS-2001
Vibrations			NOM-024-STPS-2001
Ionizing radiation			NOM-012-STPS-1999
Non-ionizing radiation			NOM-013-STPS-1993
Abnormal environmental pressures			NOM-014-STPS-2000
Thermal conditions of the medium work environment			NOM-015-STPS-2001
Ventilation			RFSHMAT Art. 99
Lighting			NOM-025-STPS-1999
Chemicals pollutants			NOM-010-STPS-1999
Identification and communication of chemical hazards			NOM-018-STPS-2000
Hazardous chemicals handling, transportation, storage and safety in chemical s. processes			NOM-005-STPS-1998 NOM-028-STPS-2004
Biological contaminants			RFSHMAT Art. 86
Ergonomic agents			RFSHMAT Art. 102
Psychological agents (psychosocial)			RFSHMAT Title III
4. Fire fighting systems			NOM-002-STPS-2000

Equipment vs. fire		NOM-100, 101, 102, 103, 104 AND 106-STPS
5. Personal protective equipment		NOM-017-STPS-2001
Footwear, helmets and protection respiratory		NOM-113, 115 AND 116-STPS
Suspended access equipment for workers at heights		NOM-009-STPS-1999
6. Electrical installations and maintenance of installations electric		NOM-023 AND 029-STPS
7. Signs, safety warnings and color codes		NOM-026-STPS-1998
8. Handling, transport and storage of materials		NOM-006-STPS-2000
9. Physical plant (buildings and premises)		NOM-001-STPS-1999
10. Order, cleanliness and services		RFSHMAT

Source: Anaya A. 2006

Working conditions

It so happens that by using the term work environment, the whole idea of a utopia enhanced with quality materials and necessary equipment in perfect conditions ceases to be real in the exercise of labor activities, according to data from the Mexican government, Mexican laws guarantee working conditions that are fundamentally related to the principle of substantive equality between women and men workers.[9]

When a person enters a company, the laws of our country establish the contracts, which are the items, the limits and the specific description of the obligations that the employee contracts with the company. In the present contract The labor conditions that the worker must have will be discussed, including the salary to be received, the type of social security acquired and, if applicable, the corresponding seniority benefits, as well as the work schedules that the person must have.

On the other hand, it is important to mention that according to a survey conducted by the Statista Research Department in April 2019, where about 40.5% said that they work in poor working conditions, however 1.2% mentioned that they have good working conditions, which undoubtedly shows the labor condition of the country, so it is important that health professionals seek strategies focused on improving conditions from public policies of health and occupational prevention respectively.[10]

Salary and hours

The main reason for entering a working day is the remuneration that the person expects to receive, in this regard, Article 82 of the Federal Labor Law provides that the company or the employer must provide a remuneration for the work performed.[9]

Since the salary is a previously established agreement between the company and the worker, which is inflexible and mandatory in our country, the minimum salary index is updated year after year, which is established by law as the lowest remuneration that the person can receive for the services and work that the person performs during working hours.

Mexican law is flexible and in many cases allows companies to calculate the salary of workers based on the services and activities they perform. It is worth mentioning that the amount that the worker receives must be greater than the minimum wage and in the case of any type of benefit, the discount will not be greater than the amount of the salary received by the worker.

The situation that employees constantly face is that of having uncertain working hours, all depending on the line of business in which the company is located, which is why there are jobs that are performed 24 hours a day, 365 days a year. such as hospitals, but others that take days off and non-working days, such as banks and schools.[9]

It is important to mention that Mexican law provides that the worker must be informed in time and, depending on the worker's condition, he/she will have the capacity to perform his/her job, this is based on articles 58 to 68 of the Federal Labor Law.

Post-pandemic time

According to data from the Mexican Institute for Competitiveness, it mentions that after the COVID 19 health crisis in Mexico, the labor area shows continuous recovery data, not only because of the creation of new jobs in different sectors, but also because of the quality of the working conditions that workers have.On the other hand, it has been demonstrated that the lodging and restaurant sectors were the ones that potentially developed their labor capacities, showing a promising recovery from the situation experienced by the pandemic.During 2022, the recovery of the labor market saw an advance in the number of jobs, it can be considered that Mexico is underemployed, but there is still a latent problem which is informality, which generates lower income perception in workers and deficiency in social security, which results in greater vulnerability in the health of the country's workers.However, studies by the Mexican Institute for Competitiveness show that the labor market has become less professionally competitive, thus devaluing the working conditions of workers as younger age groups are added to the labor force respectively.[11]

Therefore, the evolution of nursing interventions focused on occupational health has had a tenuous evolution due to the changes in the population, environmental conditions, and the development of regulatory regulations, which is why the health contingency for COVID 19 showed an increase in interest in the promotion and prevention of occupational health.The health personnel had to implement prevention strategies with the intention of preserving the health of the workers, the measures that were carried out, where the use of technologies and the development of isolation protocols in cases of illness are considered. [6]

Health care workers and occupational hazards

At present, hospital services of sanitary application that represent risks due to their complexity of application, we find services such as the blood bank, where health personnel encounter potential risks such as contact with infectious diseases such as HIV, Hepatitis B, among others.[12]

Evidently the contagion by contact with blood and other biological fluids that arise in contact with infected patients, especially to health care workers in the emergency services in the same way these services very often present situations in which the care provided is performed in complex conditions and that undoubtedly expose health care personnel, since they do not take the necessary precautions to be injured or infected. [13]

It is necessary to pay attention to the facilities in which health care workers work. In fact, labor statistics in the United States indicate that 38.2% of injuries to health care workers were the result of falls and slips, as well as injuries associated with poor body ergonomics when providing the necessary care in hospital institutions.[14]

In short, it is possible to prevent harm to healthcare personnel and constant exposure to risks, for this reason hospital institutions should work to provide the necessary personal protective equipment to carry out their work in a professional manner, however in recent years occupational risks focused on the mental state have increased considerably, especially with the emergence of the COVID 19 pandemic.

Conclusions

With regard to occupational hazards at present, there is a compromising scenario, so it is necessary to pay special attention to health assessment protocols to prevent them to a greater extent.Sometimes workers generate inaccurate and rather utopian health perspectives in the labor scenarios in which they are applied, which is why, depending on the labor category, employers will have to apply the rules for their protection.On the other hand, it is identified that, in the area of health, occupational risks have an exponential growth due to factors external to the workers, where there are deficiencies and lack of communication, generating serious damage to the health of workers and creating losses for employers.Finally, health care workers must work with the necessary precautions, preserving the quality of care provided, regardless of the circumstances in which personal protective equipment and supplies are used.

References

1. Alberto. A. Alonso. Risk Management. [Internet]. 1st ed. Alonso AA, editor. Vol. 1, Ediciones Anticipar. Autonomous City of Buenos Aires : Anticipar; 2018 [cited 2022 Jun 17]. Available from: https://www.ancient-origins.es/noticias- generallplaces-ancient-africa/the-millenary-unknown-art-rupestrian-egyptian- 003558.
2. ISO 18001. Occupational risk: definition and basic concepts [Internet]. Iso Tools. 2015 [cited 2022 Jun 17, 2022]. Available from: https://www.isotools.org/2015/09/10/riesgo-laboral-definicion-y-conceptos-basicos/
3. Félix Urbaneja Arrúe, Arantza Lijó Bilbao, Jose Ignacio Cabrerizo Benito, Jasone Idiazabal Garmendia, Ana Rosa Zubía Ortiz de Guinea, Arrate Padilla Magunacelaya. Epidemiological surveillance at work. Guide for the implementation of collective surveillance by prevention services [Internet].
OSLAN. Basque Institute of Occupational Safety and Health, editor. Vol. 1, OSALAN. Barakaldo. Vasc0: Eusko Jauralaritza; 2015 [cited 2022 Jun 17]. Available at: https://www.osalan.euskadi.eus/libro/vigilancia-epidemiologica-en- el-trabajo-guia-para-la-implantacion-de-la-impletacion-de-la-vigilancia-collectiva-por-parte-de-los- servicios-de-prevencion/s94-osa9996/en/adjuntos/guia_vigilancia_epidemiologica_2015.pdf.
4. (Decent work resource platform for sustainable development). 23 Conditions of work [Internet]. International labour organization. 2016 [cited 2016 Jun 17, 2022]. Available from: https://www.ilo.org/global/topics/dw4sd/themes/working-conditions/lang-- en/index.htm.
5. CEOE. State Foundation for the Prevention of Occupational Risks. Mexico - Prevención de Riesgos Laborales [Internet]. Ministry of labor, migration and social security . 2019 [cited 2022 Jun 17, 2022]. Available from: https://prl.ceoe.es/informacion/prl-en-el-mundo/mexico/
6. Arturo Juárez-García, Elena Hernández-Mendoza. Nursing interventions in occupational health. Rev Enferm Inst Mex Seguro Soc [Internet]. 2010 [cited 2022 June 17];23-9. Available from: https://www.medigraphic.com/pdfs/enfermeriaimss/eim-2010/eim101e.pdf
7. Secretary of Public Education. Prevention of occupational hazards [Internet]. Colegio de bachilleres . 2018 [cited 2018 Jun 29, 2022]. Available from: https://huelladigital.cbachilleres.edu.mx/secciones/docs/guias/laboral/6to-semestre/prevencion-de- riesgos-de-trabajo.pdf.
8. Anaya A. Diagnóstico de seguridad e higiene del trabajo listados de verificación basados en la normatividad mexicana occupational health and safety diagnostic verification lists based on mexican regulations. 2006 [cited June 29, 2006].2022]; Available from: www.e-gnosis.udg.mx/vol4/art3www.cusur.udg.mx
9. Government of Mexico. Condiciones de Trabajo | Tus derechos Laborales [Internet]. gob.mx. 2015 [cited 2015 June 17, 2022]. Available from: https://www.gob.mx/derechoslaborales/articulos/condiciones-de-trabajo
10. Statista. Working conditions of workers in Mexico [Internet]. Statista Research Department. 2019 [cited June 17, 2022]. Available from: https://es.statista.com/estadisticas/1124859/condiciones-laborales-trabajadores-

mexico/

11. Mexican Institute for Competitiveness A.C. Employment recovery in 2021 faced with insufficiency, informality and working poverty [Internet]. imco.org.mx. 2021 [cited 2022 June 17]. Available from: https://imco.org.mx/wp-content/uploads/2022/02/El-mercado-laboral-de-México-al- cierre-del-2021_Documento_20220225.docx-1.pdf.

12. Public Health Institute of Chile. Guide for the evaluation of security risks in hospital establishments [Internet]. Instituto de Salud. Vol. 1. Chile: Occupational Safety Section; 2016 [cited 2016 Jun 17, 2022]. Available from: https://www.ispch.cl/sites/default/files/D034-PR-500-02-001 Guia eval eval riesgos seguridad est hospitalarios.pdf.

13. Jiménez Paneque R, Pavés Carvajal JR. Occupational diseases and risks in emergency department workers: literature review and approach to Chile. Medwave [Internet]. on August 31, 2015 [cited 2022 June 29];15(07):e6239. Available from: /link.cgi/Medwave/Revision/RevisionTopics/6239.act

14. CDC - Health care workers - NIOSH health and safety topics [Internet]. [cited 2022 Jun 29, 2022]. Available from: https://www.cdc.gov/spanish/niosh/topics/trabajadores.html

CHAPTER 4

EMPLOYEE HEALTH EFFICIENCY RESOURCE NETWORK

Aurora Sierra Canto ** Patricia Carolina Cruz Heredia* William Alberto Huertas Marrufo* Patricia Carolina Cruz Heredia* William Alberto Huertas Marrufo* Patricia Carolina Cruz Heredia* William Alberto Huertas Marrufo

Traditional prevention, risk and hazard control tools remain effective when properly applied, but need to be complemented by strategies designed to anticipate, identify, assess and control the risks arising from the constant adaptation to a rapidly changing world of work.

International Labor Organization, 2009.

Introduction

The following chapter presents a glimpse of the current panorama of actions, regulations, as well as regulatory institutions that exist in terms of occupational health for the efficiency of workers' health both nationally and internationally to ensure the safe performance of their activities.Fundamentally, occupational health refers to the physical, social and psychological circumstances of employees and which condition their ability to perform their duties and/or activities adequately, and seeks to promote well-being and prevent as well as reduce accidents at work.[1]

It is relevant to mention that worker protection is related to employee productivity; according to the Ministry of Labor and Social Welfare, in Mexico, in the 2012-2016 period, on average, each year 532

*Student of the Bachelor's Degree in Nursing. Autonomous University of Yucatan

**Career Professor. Faculty of Nursing. Autonomous University of Yucatan

1,550 work-related accidents and, while on the job, 8,830 people became ill as a result of their work and 1,406 died while performing their work or as a result of it, at the Mexican Social Security Institute (IMSS).[2]

For an employer, the health of its workers is essential, because if they have health, well-being and dignified treatment, their performance will be better and therefore the employer will obtain higher profits, so the network of resources that are used to improve occupational health is essential and are of great importance for both workers and bosses.This network of resources includes regulatory institutions, as well as international and national laws and regulations, and is responsible for establishing and enforcing occupational health and safety strategies.These organizations include the International Labor Organization (ILO) and the World Health Organization (WHO), the Pan American Health Organization at the global level, as well as various trade unions such as the Confederación de Trabajadores de México at the national level. Mexico is a member country of the World Health Organization and the International Labor Organization; therefore, one of its obligations is to guarantee compliance with and respect for human rights and to protect workers by creating laws, regulations and agreements to safeguard human rights in labor institutions. The regulations related to Occupational Health and Safety are extensive, however, the basis of such regulations is the Political Constitution of the United Mexican States, followed by the various norms and laws created to improve the aspects related to the health and safety of employees.

International panorama

At the international level, there are regulatory organizations to ensure the safety of workers, including the International Labor Organization (ILO), the World Health Organization (WHO) and the Pan American Health Organization (PAHO).[1]

Thus, these organizations, in an effort to improve the quality of occupational health in partner countries, have promoted initiatives to get governments to create or modify public policies on occupational safety and health so that employers allocate investment capital to strengthen the prevention of occupational accidents and diseases.[1]

For its part, the World Health Organization (WHO), based on the World Health Assembly entitled "Workers' Health: A Plan of Action "[3], establishes multiple strategies for member countries to make efforts to improve the scope and quality of health care provided to workers, including small businesses and the informal economic sector, among these recommendations:

• Provide and reinforce the training given to health workers (general practitioners, nurses and community health workers) so that they are able to provide their services focused and adapted to the occupational health context.

• To expand the coverage of services focused on occupational health, as well as to improve the quality of these services in both large and medium-sized companies, with special emphasis on the evaluation and reduction of occupational risks, health promotion, as well as the surveillance and maximization of the safety of the work environment.

• Create referral and counter-referral channels between occupational health services and primary care institutions, in order to expedite and facilitate care for workers who suffer from a chronic degenerative disease or occupational illness and need to use this service, with the aim of ensuring their return to work after the period of illness.

• Create workplace health strategies, algorithms and protocols to improve employee health without the need to rely entirely on health care providers and services.

• Training of health personnel by the institutions on occupational health issues upon entry and during the performance of their activities in the hospitals.

Likewise, the International Labor Organization (ILO) in its constitution establishes the basis that employees must be protected against possible illnesses and accidents that may occur in the work environment. All of the ILO's stipulations on occupational safety and health provide governments, employers and employees with the necessary tools to create methods to ensure maximum occupational safety.[4]

It is for this reason that in its effort to ensure a safe and healthy work environment for employees, it establishes that partner countries should focus their efforts on creating national Occupational Safety and Health (OSH) systems. According to the International Labor Organization 2020, this system should consist of several elements, including legislation and enforcement mechanisms, as well as training and an information network. The system should be continuously improved through the formulation and implementation of national OSH programs as outlined in the Promotional Framework for Occupational Safety and Health Convention (No. 187) and its accompanying Recommendation (No. 197).[5]

ILO [6] establishes that OSH laws and regulations must comply with the following items:

• General duty of employers to protect the physical and mental health of workers.

• Requirements for the adoption of OSH preventive measures (policies; risk assessment; protocols and procedures; training; etc.).

• Mechanisms for filing complaints.
• Protection against retaliation.
• Penalties, remediation and compensation.

Finally, the Pan American Health Organization (PAHO) is an international organization that seeks to guarantee the health of workers. Its main task is to provide technical advice to member countries in the Americas region in order to promote the development and continuous improvement of work environments to make them healthy and safe. PAHO seeks to effectively prevent any type of harm, injury, illness and death related to work or the environment in which work is performed, as well as making efforts to respond to global, regional and national priorities in occupational health and safety.[7]

PAHO's work to improve occupational health also includes providing technical assistance to governments and employers to promote workers' access to quality health care, as well as to achieve the following objectives:

1. Strengthen regulatory standards and health sector leadership in member countries.

2. Promote the health of workers, as well as the creation and maintenance of workplaces that are safe, healthy and productive.

3. Prevent and catalog illnesses, accidents and fatalities that occur in the work environment.

4. Ensure access to universal health care.

5. In addition, to pay attention to critical economic sectors due to their impact on the health of the general population. [7]

In addition, PAHO is working on the Plan of Action on Workers' Health 2015-2025, which seeks to respond to the national, regional and global priorities defined by PAHO/WHO for workers' health, as well as to contribute to the achievement of the Sustainable Development Goals (SDGs), in particular SDG 1, SDG 3 and SDG 8. [7]

As for labor standards, they serve as essential tools for the governments of different countries to create and establish labor laws in accordance with international standards and to protect the human rights of workers.[2]

The International Labor Organization[2] states that the most important treaties at the international level are:

- C 155 on occupational safety and health (1981)
- Promotes the creation, implementation and periodic evaluation of specific OSH-related standards by Member States.

- C 161 on occupational health services (1985)
- It provides for the establishment of health services in public or private workplaces, which provide preventive services and advice to employers and workers.

- "All workers shall be informed of the health risks involved in their work." (Article 13)

- C 187 on the Promotional Framework for Occupational Safety and Health (2006)
- It aims to promote a culture of prevention with a view to the progressive achievement of a safe and healthy work environment. It requires the development of national policies, systems and programs.

- "Each Member shall promote and encourage the right of workers to a safe and healthy working environment". (Article 3, numeral 2)

National Overview

At the national level, the most important regulatory agency is the Ministry of Labor and Social Welfare (STPS), which is responsible for enforcing labor policies and moderating compliance with workers' rights through various strategies such as adequate training of employees, establishment of channels for social dialogue between employees and employers, as well as the right to unionize. [8]

In the years following the creation of the STPS, other organizations responsible for regulating occupational health have been established, known as workers' unions, which are alliances formed between various unions and labor and non-labor groups to achieve common objectives.[9]

The Confederation of Mexican Workers (CTM) is an organization made up mainly of workers and proletarian classes, which from the beginning has been in charge of fighting injustice and bringing about a change in society, eliminating exploitation and inequalities in the distribution of capital. [10]

Some of the actions carried out by this confederation to promote the health of its members are: [10]

- To avoid the exploitation of people, to improve the living conditions, health, employment and remuneration of workers.

- Providing a wage that gives workers a decent living
- Providing workers with comfortable, hygienic housing
- To favor the consolidation and strengthening of the Mexican Social Security Institute as the highest social security body in Mexico.

On the other hand, there are other union organizations that also seek to reinforce compliance with regulations in the workplace, in order to create a dignified and safe working environment for workers. Some of these existing organizations are:

- The Sindicato Nacional De Trabajadores Del Seguro Social (SNTSS) 2018-2024 has the mission to safeguard the rights of the workers of the Mexican Social Security Institute. Additionally, to contribute with all that is necessary to strengthen the institute and continue to be the maximum provider of health services. [11]

- The Sindicato Nacional de Trabajadores de la Secretaría de Salud (SNTSA), which seeks the study, improvement and defense of the labor interests of its members, under the terms established by law and supplementary legal provisions. [12]

In Mexico, the main basis of the regulatory framework related to OSH is Article 123 of the Political Constitution of the United Mexican States, together with the rules, laws and regulations, are useful to provide adequate protection to workers. One of the authorities in charge of verifying compliance with the regulations at the national level is the Secretaría del Trabajo y Previsión Social (Ministry of Labor and Social Welfare). [2]

The Political Constitution of the United Mexican States has the scope of protecting and guaranteeing human rights, the exercise and practice of a profession or employment, as well as the right to dignified or decent work. [2]

In addition to the Political Constitution, one of the components that regulates the right to work is the Federal Labor Law (LFT), guiding labor relations, favoring decent work and establishing a balance with the standards developed. [2]

Likewise, the Federal Occupational Safety and Health Regulation establishes the OSH provisions, in order to have the conditions to prevent occupational risks and guarantee workers the right to perform their activities in an environment that ensures their life and health, in accordance with the provisions of the LFT. [2]

The objective of these regulations and legal instruments is to guarantee the protection of health and life in the workplace, to promote dignified and healthy work environments, and to strengthen a culture of prevention in the workplace. [2]

Additionally in Mexico, the National Development Plan, in its 2019-2024 edition, establishes the objective "2. Guarantee employment, education, health and welfare" which mentions that it will be given in accordance with the creation of new jobs, increased investment in infrastructure and health services, along with the development of regional programs that favor the population. [13]

Some of the strategies established prior to the National Development Plan were "Promote decent work" and "Improve the systems and procedures for the protection of workers' rights", which sought to promote decent employment for citizens, promote the importance of respect for human rights, favor the elimination of child labor, and encourage the development of a culture of social justice. the participation of labor organizations to improve their health and safety policies in the institutions. [2]

According to the Mexican Institute of Social Security (2018), some actions are established that are carried out to guarantee the health of the working population, these are: [14]

• Achieve higher levels of social security coverage by incorporating a greater number of workers, mainly those in the informal sector, into the Social Security system.

• Strengthen the process of education and training in Occupational Safety and Health, both for employers and workers, in order to influence a culture of prevention at all levels.

Conclusions

Within the framework of the above considerations, international and national regulatory organizations play a fundamental role in occupational health, since they establish strategies, regulations, laws and agreements in order to provide a safe working environment that favors the health of workers.

However, even with the existence of these organizations and regulations, some companies and workplaces do not respect what they establish, or do not make the appropriate modifications to the regulations in the establishments or simply ignore the recommendations and strategies because employers are not willing to allocate funds to protect the occupational health of employees since they see it as an economic loss.Therefore, due to the poor working conditions in which employees find themselves, there is a decrease in their performance and efficiency, although many bosses do not give importance to occupational health and the strategies established to improve it, if they were more aware of the needs of their workers, they would realize that when a person feels safe, has health, welfare and dignified treatment, their job performance will be higher and therefore employers will receive greater benefits. In view of this situation, it is necessary to strengthen the supervision of compliance with national regulations to fortify the safety of workers in the workplace, as well as to provide information about existing regulations related to occupational health and safety, since most workers do not know about the existence of the regulations and the institutions in charge, and therefore do not enforce their rights to a dignified and safe working environment.A fundamental strategy in terms of occupational health would be to invite the population to be informed about the rights to which they have access when working in an institution and the safety criteria that employers must implement, awareness campaigns should be created through digital media and communication so that employees know their rights and can demand an improvement in their work environments.As a last point, it is important to mention the importance of establishing proper communication among workers so that they can organize themselves and thus demand dignified treatment, express their ideas and opinions about their occupational health needs, and establish a good relationship with employers to create agreements that favor both parties.Good organization among workers is fundamental, as it helps to encourage employers to comply with the rights and obligations established by organizations and regulations, as well as access to health services and improve their working conditions to have a better quality of life.

References

1. Fagua G, De Hoz Y, Jaimes J. Occupational safety and health management system: a review from emergency plans. Multidisciplinary Scientific Journal [Internet]. 2018 [Accessed 2022 Jun 06]; 3(1): 23-29. Available from: https://latinjournal.org/index.php/ipsa/article/view/920/700
2. Secretaría Del Trabajo Y Previsión Social. Safety and Health at Work in Mexico: Advances, challenges and challenges. [Internet]. Mexico: Government of Mexico; 2017.
[Accessed 2022 Jun 14]. Available at: https://www.gob.mx/cms/uploads/attachment/file/279153/Libro-Seguridad_y_salud_en_el_trabajo_en_Me_xico.
Advances retos_y_desafios Digital_.pdf.
3. World Health Organization. Workers' health protection [Internet]. United States of America: WHO; 2017 [Accessed 2022 Jun 04]. Available from: https://www.who.int/es/news-room/fact-sheets/detail/protecting- workers'-health.
4. International Labour Organization. Occupational safety and health [Internet]. United States of America; ILO; 2022 [Accessed 2022 Jun 04]. Available from: https://www.ilo.org/global/standards/subjects-covered-by-international-labour-standards/occupational-safety-and-health/lang--en/index.htm.
5. International Labour Organization. National occupational safety and health systems and programs [Internet]. United States of America; ILO; 2020 [Accessed 2022 Jun 04]. Available from: https://www.ilo.org/global/topics/safety- and-health-at-work/areasofwork/national-occupational-safety-and-health-systems- and-programmes/lang--en/index.htm.
6. International Labour Organization. PPT Presentatión "Safe and healthy work environments, free from violence and harassment" [Internet]. United States of America; ILO; 2020 [Accessed 2022 Jun 04].Available from: https://www.ilo.org/wcmsp5/groups/public/---ed_protect/---protrav/---safework/documents/presentation/wcms_751909.pptx.
7. Pan American Health Organization. Workers' health [Internet]. United States of

America; PAHO/WHO; 2020 [Accessed 2022 Jun 04]. Available from: https://www.paho.org/es/temas/salud-trabajadores

8. Secretaría de Trabajo y Previsión Social [Internet]. Mexico; STPS: [Accessed 2022 Jun 05]. Available at: https://www.gob.mx/stps

9. HMONG. Community trade unionism. [Internet]; 2017. [Accessed 2022 Jun 14]. Available from: https://hmong.es/wiki/Community_unionism.

10. Confederation of Mexican Workers. Confederation of Workers of Mexico. [Online]; 2020. [Accessed 2022 Jun 14]. Available from: https://ctmoficial.org/principios-2/.

11. National Executive Committee of the National Union of Social Security Workers. Sindicato Nacional De Trabajadores Del Seguro Social. [Internet]; 2018. [Accessed 2022 Jun 14]. Available from: https://sntss.org.mx/quienes-somos.

12. National Union of Health Secretariat Workers. Objectives [Internet]. Mexico: SNTSA; [Accessed 2022 Jun 05]. Available at: https://sindicatodesalud.org.mx/?page_id=32

13. Ministry of the Interior. Diario Oficial de la Federación. [Internet]; 2019. [Accessed 2022 Jun 14]. Available from: https://www.dof.gob.mx/nota_detalle.php?codigo=5565599&fecha=12/07/2019#gsc.tab=0.

14. Mexican Institute of Social Security. Institutional Program of the Mexican Institute of Social Security 2014-2018. [Internet].; 2018. [Accessed 2022 Jun 14]. Available from: https://www.imss.gob.mx/sites/all/statics/pdf/PIIMSS_2014-2018_FINAL_230414.pdf.

CHAPTER 5

OCCUPATIONAL HAZARDS OF HEALTH PERSONNEL

Janet Carolina Negrón Espadas** Aurora Sierra Canto**
Daniel Eduardo Trujeque Córdoba* Estefany Alejandra Ku Noh* Estefany Alejandra
Ku Noh* Daniel Eduardo Trujeque Córdoba* Estefany Alejandra Ku Noh
"Accident prevention should not be considered as a matter of legislation, but as a duty to human beings, and as a reason of economic sense."

Werner Von Siemens (1892)

Introduction

Work is that which requires time and people for the production of a good or service. In the case of health personnel, it is performed when they provide various services for the prevention of disease, cure or recovery of people's health.In the same sense, health is a human right and a source of economic and social development for the country. In Mexico, public institutions have approximately 650,000 health care workers (2007). About 171,000 are physicians in contact with patients; 223,000 are nurses, and 85,000 are paramedical personnel and personnel involved in auxiliary diagnostic and treatment services, and 182,000 are health personnel classified as "other".

*Student of the Bachelor's Degree in Nursing. Autonomous University of Yucatan

**Career Professor. Faculty of Nursing. Autonomous University of Yucatan

It should be noted that, according to the World Health Organization (WHO), occupational health is that multidisciplinary activity that promotes and protects the health of workers, however, health personnel are exposed to occupational hazards. In fact, occupational risk is a condition that can cause progressive or direct damage to health personnel, whether physical or mental.It is erroneously believed that health personnel are not at risk of suffering any harm during their work because they are the ones who perform the care, but the reality is different. It is often not given enough importance for the implementation of occupational risk prevention. Specifically in the health care area, all workers are vulnerable to occupational hazards to a greater or lesser extent; however, some documents show that nursing and anesthesiology personnel are subject to greater risks; however, this should not exclude the other professionals and technicians who make up the health care team.As previously mentioned, there are different risks, including: biological risks such as punctures, cuts, infectious diseases; chemical risks such as anesthetic gases, disinfectants, sterilization liquids, handling of drugs and the use of electrocautery; physical risks such as noise, ionizing radiation and non-ionizing radiation; ergonomic risks such as bad posture, long periods of time in one position, among others (1).

In healthcare personnel, it has been shown that the greatest risk is present with acute or chronic infections. That is why it is important to recognize occupational hazards and know where they are generated. In order to create and implement preventive measures. In this case, biosafety is a key element, since it represents the set of protocols, principles, standards or processes to analyze health and environmental risks.This chapter contains the main occupational hazards of health personnel, in order to make them known and create a source of information for future readers. Above all, to give them visibility and importance for the creation of strategies, having as a result, the gradual decrease of these risks. (2)

Situation analysis

According to the WHO, health is a state of complete physical, mental and social well-being, and not merely the absence of disease or infirmity. In the case of work, it is that physical or intellectual activity that is accompanied by a purpose and is economically remunerated. On the other hand, occupational health is responsible for promoting and protecting the health of workers.It should be noted that occupational health risk appears with the recognition, implicit or explicit, of the right to physical integrity and health, something that appears in the High Middle Ages and the Renaissance. Occupational health risks are defined as situations and behaviors that cannot be accepted because of their harmful consequences for workers (3).

Occupational safety is necessary to ensure the quality of life of workers, so health risks in the work area must be identified. This requires a trained multidisciplinary team.In this same sense, health professionals are at high risk of accidentally contracting infectious diseases during their work in health care. Direct patient care with body fluids and the cultivation or sampling of infectious microorganisms during laboratory studies are the main factors that produce an increased risk, and therefore adversely affect the quality of life of these employees, due to the unsafe conditions of the job (4).

Therefore, it is essential to identify occupational hazards in order to control the situations that generate them and to define the appropriate bases for prevention and promotion that favor the well-being of workers. In the case of the health sector, biosecurity measures are appropriate for the management of occupational hazards that have an impact on the vulnerability of workers.In general terms, the occupational risk factors to which health professionals are immersed alter each type of personnel in a different way, this is because the level of exposure of each is different from the other, i.e., the occupational vulnerability of nurses will be different from that of chemists, doctors, etc.Nursing professionals are especially at risk, due to their close and permanent contact with the people under their care. This is followed by laboratory personnel and cleaning personnel who handle biological samples, even though their contact with patients is reduced. Thus, occupational risk in health sector workers can be divided into: (4)

Biological hazards

Biological occupational hazard is understood as any infection, allergy or toxicity caused by microorganisms (including genetically modified microorganisms, cell cultures and human endoparasites) that a worker may contract". Biological hazards are produced by microorganisms, such as cell cultures, parasites, tissues and organs of the human body, capable of producing any infection or allergy and these can trigger damage to the health of workers. (1, 5)

Chemical hazards

It is the unmoderated exposure to chemical agents, which can produce acute or chronic deterioration in the professional's health. This is established by the toxicity of the substances used in the hospital area and the material of the product and its route of application. This type of risk can cause irritation of the larynx and pharynx, lung, asthma, dyspnea, wheezing, burning eyes and diseases such as conjunctivitis. Cleaning personnel are the most affected and should be the target of major prevention and health promotion strategies to control and reduce the possibility of incidence. (1)

In the surgical area, electrocautery is the most commonly used by physicians because it allows invasive surgical techniques to be carried out satisfactorily. It has been determined that the smoke it produces causes damage to health such as: chromosomal alterations and the development of cancer (1) (2).

Psychological risks

Psychological factors include those cognitive, affective and behavioral processes that can affect the professional's work performance, causing anxiety, depression, Burnout syndrome, stress, etc.

In the hospital environment, due to the nature of the area, it involves an intense workload, professional wear and tear, physical and emotional fatigue, resulting in high levels of stress, which is one of the main psychological conditions affecting human beings in their working life (1).

Physical risks

In the hospital environment, electromagnetic radiation (UV rays, gamma rays, X-rays) is used. This not only harms the professional who is in charge of the application of X-rays, but also those who are close to this area (1).

Ergonomic risks

Ergonomic risks establish any situation that may affect the professional's comfort at work, this is defined as: the relationship between the work environment and the employees; such as bad posture, sudden and abrupt movements and musculoskeletal disorders.A physical effort of greater capacity of response than the person who exerts it can produce, causes the development of work-related musculoskeletal injuries (1).

Situation of health sector workers vis-à-vis COVID-19

Recent reports by the World Health Organization (WHO) indicate that more than 22,000 workers in this sector have been infected with the SARS-CoV-2 virus and hundreds of health professionals have died in different countries. These figures may be subject to underreporting due to limitations in data collection and real-time recording, as well as inconsistent reporting due to the collapse of some information systems. (6)

Recent research conducted in China and the United States indicates that health care workers are more vulnerable to illness during their workday, and that their risk is greater when they work in areas where they are not at work. This is closely related to their perception of the possible route of contagion. The WHO and some studies on the subject report that risk factors for occupational exposure include low or absent availability of personal protective equipment (PPE), late diagnosis of users, long working hours, non-compliance with infection control protocols and inadequate management of the respiratory tract. The means of transmission of SARS-CoV-2 is mainly by droplets and fomites; therefore, standard measures for the reduction and spread of the virus mainly promote proper hand washing and the use of barriers and respiratory protection. However, these measures have been difficult to comply with due to various situations at work, the main one being the overcrowding of services and the unavailability of PPE. (7)

Administrative measures

In hospitals, risk assessments must be carried out in order to know the hazards of the workplace for health personnel. This is why it is important to optimally and effectively manage the health and safety of a hospital, especially to implement measures and policies to ensure the safety of workers.

Infection control policies

Currently, infection prevention and control policies were determined by the WHO and multiple regional health institutions; therefore, by taking these as a structural basis, guidelines have been created for the use, prevention and control of the new virus, which are constantly updated as new scientific evidence appears (8,9).

The use of an infection control program in institutions allows for rapid action in the event of emergencies or situations related to risky health care. This instrument should be used at the various levels of health care. At the intrahospital level, the creation of the Infection Control Program is the reference point for activities in this direction. It should be made up of a trained multidisciplinary group; it should also include with the participation of the institution's authorities, specialized personnel and experts from the administrative area, to establish rapid, timely and effective communication with those responsible for the occupational health departments and the administration. This team will direct and guide the use of policies that protect the needs of the health professional and the institution (8,9).

The integration of the team is essential for making immediate decisions on identified risks and in the event of threats or adverse events. As part of the initial activities, the team will establish a budget to maintain and sustain the program as required. These policies suggest that within the multidisciplinary group, a qualified person (health professional) should be established to work on a temporary or permanent basis, depending on the complexity of the health institution. However, it is likely that the current situation will require exclusive dedication or the support of a support staff. These health personnel will help design, execute and supervise the Infection Control Plan (ICP) based on the risk diagnosis carried out and determine all the policies and guidelines that respond to the needs of the employees and the facility.Because of this, these policies should not only be oriented to health personnel but also to cleaning and maintenance personnel. The instrument should establish the strategies recommended by the health authorities; and should include adequate and continuous training, as well as continuous updating on the epidemiology of SARS-CoV-2 and its standard precautions, which will be implemented with all personnel working in the health institution.Surveillance and control of personnel suspected of having COVID-19 or at risk of contracting the disease is essential to reduce exposure to the infection among health professionals. Communication should be continuous and effective with personnel when COVID-19 infection is suspected and isolation of the worker from factors that imply a greater risk that could deteriorate his or her physical or mental integrity. The occupational health department should develop or adopt tools that facilitate the evaluation and establishment of the professional's risk profile (9).

The environmental and infrastructure aspects are those measures aimed at complying with ventilation, space distribution, engineering and disinfection measures, depending on the development and control of administrative measures (10).

Hospital reconversion

With regard to the distribution of spaces in the hospital setting, it is of great importance that facilities oriented to the care of users with suspected or confirmed COVID-19 have exclusive and separate areas, such as areas for the use of health care personnel, triage areas, and areas for the care of mild to moderate cases other than those for severe and critical cases. They should be marked with exclusive and isolated access points for the exit and entry of users and health professionals; this will reduce the risk of cross-infection; they should also have easily accessible paths for the transfer of users when their condition improves or worsens; basic services such as water, waste disposal and solid and adequate infrastructure should be included. Given the lack of capacity in hospitals, some countries used their specialized areas for the care of critical patients. In order to comply, they made modifications to their physical and material infrastructure; in addition to implementing training for their personnel. This has a great impact on those health systems that do not have sufficient resources and support from national authorities (10,11). (10,11)

Likewise, isolation of individuals is another key strategy. In healthcare institutions with sufficient resources, the use of an exclusive restroom for confirmed users is an appropriate strategy. However, this is not feasible in hospital settings where patient demand exceeds the number of rooms or in countries whose hospitals are severely cramped for space. For this purpose, the use of hospitalization areas with good ventilation can be shared by many users with the same diagnosis and severity of the disease, maintaining a separation of at least one meter between patient beds (11).

Ventilation

On the other hand, in the different results obtained from the studies done so far have been concluded, this is due to the aerosol transmission of SARS-CoV2. Specialists mention that, if this is the case, it does not exclude contagion, when speaking as well as breathing. In this regard, Van Doremalen et al (2020) found that, under controlled conditions, SARS-CoV2 can remain for three hours maintaining its infectious capacity in aerosols, these conditions can be alarming for the infection of other people, in closed environments that do not have adequate ventilation, so ventilation must be adequate in high-risk places.In places with scarce resources, natural ventilation is one of the easiest and easiest to implement, because it is achieved by keeping windows or air intakes open so that cross ventilation is achieved.In a hospital environment, natural ventilation with a flow rate of 60L/S per patient is required; on the other hand, in high-risk areas or where procedures that generate aerosols are performed, mechanical ventilation is adequate for these situations and has a flow rate of 160S/L per user, achieving a negative pressure of 12 air exchanges per hour. (12, 13)

Disinfection

Another essential activity in the contingency for the care of infected users is the hygiene of spaces, which must be carried out exhaustively in all the different hospital areas that are attended by the same health professional. The spread of SARS-COV-2 has been evidenced in places such as waiting rooms and common use rooms, as well as on surfaces in physical contact such as buttons, switches, handles, computers, dispensers, desks and bottles of alcohol gel. In addition, it has also been proven that the virus is capable of remaining for up to several days on some surfaces such as metal, plastic and glass, related to various environmental factors. Thus, this coronavirus is capable of being active for up to 72 hours in immobile materials such as plastic (7).

Respiratory management

Although years have passed since the beginning of the pandemic, the management of respiratory protection has not undergone major changes, because there is insufficient evidence to demonstrate the superiority of specialized respiratory protection such as KN95, N95 or FFP2/3. Currently, the WHO has recommended the universal use of respiratory protection for all workers and health professionals in all work environments. The use of N95 in places where aerosols are used, such as the intensive care unit, laboratory sampling, emergency and operating rooms, among others (7).The health authority and the manufacturers of specialized mouthguards suggest the application of tests to adjust and guarantee respiratory protection. This consists of verifying the seal of the respirator to the professional's face, as well as the choice of the correct model and size.In a study that determined the association between working conditions and access to personal protective equipment (PPE) in health professionals in the city of Lima-Peru, in which 323 virtual respondents participated, it was concluded that health professionals under 56 years of age infrequently received PPE. When they work without an employment relationship and belong to areas with little contact with COVID-19 patients, they sometimes receive a mask (14).

In view of the global lack of these mouthguards, different solution methods have been proposed, such as strategies to extend the time of use, or the use of alternative respiratory protection devices, as well as their disinfection, such as the purified air respirators or the elastomeric respirators proposed by the Center for Disease Control (CDC), both devices are reusable and have replacement filtration systems, but require a greater investment for health institutions. (7)

Conclusions

The key piece for a hospital to function properly is obviously the health personnel, as well as providing quality services to users. Therefore, it is important to prevent occupational hazards and thus generate optimal working conditions for the protection of health professionals. This chapter made it possible to analyze occupational hazards among health personnel; however, this topic merits follow-up in order to design programs and strategies aimed at all workers in health institutions. It also shows the need to carry out research focused on occupational risks in such an important population. For its part, the COVID-19 pandemic, since its appearance, generated uncertainty in the entire population and especially in the health personnel, because the physical and mental risk was affected. An important area of opportunity for improvement in health institutions is the shortage of material and personal protective equipment. That is why health personnel, especially nurses, must know the protocols of care, prevention measures to limit contagion and constant updating, all this to contribute to the physical and mental health of health workers. Among health care workers, there are risk conditions for the development of complications in case of SARS-CoV-2 infection. Most medical and nursing personnel use standard protective measures (15).

References

1. Vista de Conocimiento y exposición a riesgos laborales del personal de salud en el área quirúrgica (s/f). Edu.co. Retrieved June 16, 2022, from https://revistas.unilibre.edu.co/index.php/rc_salud_ocupa/article/view/4948/4233
2. View of biosafety standards for nursing personnel in a hospital institution (s/f). Unison.mx. Retrieved June 16, 2022, from https://biotecnia.unison.mx/index.php/biotecnia/article/view/225/182
3. Moreno Jiménez Bernardo. Psychosocial occupational factors and risks: conceptualization, history and current changes. Medicina. Seguro trab [Internet]. 2011 [cited 2022 Sep 8]; 57 (supplement 1): 4-19. Available en: http://scielo.isciii.es/scielo.php?script=sci_arttext&pid=S0465-546X2011000500002&lng=es. https://dx.doi.org/10.4321/S0465-546X2011000500002.
4. View of occupational risk in health workers in the public sector (s/f). Reciamuc.com. Retrieved June 17, 2022, from https://reciamuc.com/index.php/RECIAMUC/article/view/124/125
5. Escamilla C.D. Biological risks in the workplace. Institute of Public Health. 2023 [Internet]. [Cited September 08, 2022]: available at: https://www.ispch.cl/sites/default/files/Nota_Tecnica_N_014_Riesgos_Biologicos In_the_Labor_Environment_Use_of_Personal_Protection_Items.pdf
6. World Health Organization. Coronavirus Disease 2019 (COVID-19). Situation Report-82 [Internet]. WHO. 2020 [Cited June 17, 2022]. Available from: https://apps.who.int/iris/bitstream/hand-le/10665/331780/nCoVsitrep11Apr2020-eng.pdf?sequence=1&isA-llowed=y
7. Rodríguez-Pérez, A. U. (2022). Strategies for the prevention of COVID-19 in Health Sector workers. Revista Experiencia En Medicina Del Hospital Regional Lambayeque, 8(1) [Internet]. CDC; 2019. [Cited June 17, 2022] Available from: http://rem.hrlamb.gob.pe/index.php/REM/article/view/598/339
8. Centers for Disease Control and Prevention. Infection control in healthcare personnel: Infrastructure and routine practices for occupational infection prevention and control services [Internet]. CDC; 2019. [Cited June 17, 2022] Available from: https://www.cdc.gov/infectioncontrol/pdf/guidelines/infection-con-trol-HCP-H.pdf.
9. World Health Organization. Severe Acute Respiratory Infection (SARI) Treatment facility design. Training Modules [Internet]. WHO. 2020. [Cited June 17, 2022] Available at: https://openwho.org/courses/SARI-facilities
10. Bauchner H, Fontanarosa P, Livingston E. Conserving Supply of Perso-nal Protective Equipment-A Call for Ideas. JAMA. 2022;323(19):1911. doi:10.1001/jama.2020.477017.
11. Livingston E, Desai A, Berkwits M. Sourcing personal protective equipment during the COVID-19 pandemic. J Am Med Assoc. 2022; 2019: E1-3. doi:10.1001/jama.2020.5317.
12. Atkinson J, Chartier Y, Pessoa-Silva C, Jensen P, Li Y, Seto W-H. Natural ventilation for infection control in health-care settings. [Internet] WHO Publication/Guidelines. Geneva; 2009 [Cited June 17, 2022]. Available from:

https://www.who.int/water_sanitation_health/pu- blications/natural_ventilation/en/
13. Peters A, Chawla K, Turnbull Z. Transforming ORs into ICUs. N Engl J Med. 2020;382(19): e52. doi:10.1056/NEJMc2010853.
14. Raraz-Vidal J.G., Allpas-Gomez H.L., Raraz-Vidal O.B., Torres-Salome F.K., Cabrera-Patino W.M., Alcantara-Leyva L.M. Working conditions and personal protective equipment against COVID-19 in health personnel, Lima-Peru. 2021. [Internet]; Rev. Med. Hum. 21(2): 335-345; [Cited September 08, 2022]. Disponible en: https://www.epistemonikos.org/es/documents/88ea1b33471f9a1368c40835d09bed23b48a7857
15. Márquez-González H, Klünder-Klünder M, de la Rosa-Zamboni D, Ortega-Riosvelasco F, López-Martínez B, Jean-Tron G, Chapa-Koloffon G, Ávila- Hernández AV, Garduño-Espinosa J, Villa-Guillén M, Nieto-Zermeño J. Risk conditions in healthcare workers of a pediatric coronavirus disease center in Mexico City. [Internet], Bol Med Hosp Infant Mex. 2021 Jan 19;78(2):110-115. [Cited September 08, 2022]. Available at: https://pubmed.ncbi.nlm.nih.gov/33465059/

CHAPTER 6

WORK CONTEXT IN NURSING PROFESSIONALS IN TIMES OF COVID 19

Janet Carolina Negrón Espadas** Diana Jacqueline Figueroa Ventura* Everth Amilcar Kantún Oxte* Everth Amilcar Kantún Oxte* Diana Jacqueline Figueroa Ventura* Everth Amilcar Kantún Oxte
The nurse's sole function is to help the sick or healthy individual.

Virginia Henderson.

Introduction

At the end of 2019, multiple cases of patients hospitalized for pneumonia and respiratory failure of unknown origin were reported in the city of Wuhan, China, where a high percentage of patients had even more severe complications. In early January 2020, the Chinese Ministry of Health had already identified a new coronavirus as a possible etiology, however, the cause was quickly identified and also rapidly spread in China and Asia, as well as other parts of the world.(1)

It was in February of the same year that the World Health Organization (WHO) named this pathology as COVID-19 (Coronavirus Disease 19) which is currently known to be an asymptomatic respiratory disease or with symptoms common to the common flu, from mild, in the initial, influenza or viral response phase, to severe with symptoms of pneumonia in the inflammatory or pulmonary phase and the possibility of progression to the hyperinflammatory or systemic phase with complications such as Severe Acute Respiratory Syndrome (SARS) and/or multi-organ dysfunction that can be fatal. COVID 19 is caused by the SARS-COV-2 virus, belonging to the coronavirus family (2).

*Student of the Bachelor's Degree in Nursing. Autonomous University of Yucatan

**Career Professor. Faculty of Nursing. Autonomous University of Yucatan

With confirmed cases of COVID-19 almost worldwide, WHO and the Pan American Health Organization (PAHO) on March 11, 2020 had recognized the pandemic status as this virus is highly contagious and is transmitted rapidly through coughing or respiratory secretions, by close contact, as well as through contaminated hands and/or fomites that come in contact with the mouth, nose and eyes(3).

Due to the sudden appearance and rapid spread caused by the virus, the need for hospitalization of patients was so high that hospitals were overloaded, revealing all the previously existing needs of the same as well as the increase in the lack of material, human and financial resources of many of the public health services, Among the problems with shortage of basic material resources such as lack of gloves, sterile gauze and even important material such as Personal Protective Equipment (PPE) for the health team, on the other hand, also the hospitals denoted their structural problems, previously already existing in terms of capacity and functionality. All these problems related to care management affect both the patients who receive care, as well as the health personnel who struggle to perform their work effectively and efficiently, despite the high risk to their health and integrity.(4,5)

Throughout this chapter, we will analyze the work context of nursing professionals in times of COVID 19, personnel who have been in the front line in the fight against pandemics that threaten health worldwide, demonstrating their compassion, courage and bravery when providing care. The analysis will be based on four aspects: the role, occupational health, mental health and the perception of nursing professionals.

Nursing Role during the COVID 19 Pandemic

Health personnel during this pandemic have been a pillar in the progress of hospital and community care, since they have remained at the forefront in providing care to those who are hospitalized, operating from triage and first contact to isolation areas to each person with symptoms, and also providing care and using preventive methods to protect patients who are hospitalized for reasons other than COVID 19, who are also essential to continue caring for because they became part of the risk groups. On the other hand, at the community level, nurses provide health education and guidance to stay at home and comply with social distancing, as well as sharing truthful, consistent and updated information to dispel myths and reduce the population's anxiety.For this reason, safety protocols were established to reduce the risk of cross-infection between patients and health professionals, taking into account measures such as the creation of a scale of health professionals to identify people with respiratory symptoms, the formation of a Rapid Response Team, the establishment of shifts for nursing teams in the care scales for patients with symptoms or suspected COVID 19, which gave good results, adding collaboration to social isolation and the reduction of crowds in closed places to avoid a greater number of infections.Therefore, the nursing staff has made innovations in health education, providing the population with safe support in terms of information and self-care during the pandemic, following up on safety measures, carrying out health promotion to reduce the dissemination of false information and thus contributing to the insecurity of the population.These strategies reduce risk behaviors and, therefore, contagion, thus reducing overcrowding in hospitalization areas. As part of these strategies, the promotion of home quarantine and isolation for at least 14 days was implemented, and explanatory information was shared on new terms, such as The vaccination scheme was subsequently introduced, for which the nursing staff has also been the basis for orientation on the benefits and proven information on vaccination, Likewise, this vaccination period has brought new challenges for nurses due to the reluctance to the vaccine because of the population's misinformation; however, doubts have been dispelled with a greater number of acceptance, which guarantees greater coverage in the protection against the SARS COV 2 virus.(4)

Occupational health in the hospital setting during the COVID 19 pandemic.

In-hospital SARS VOC 2 infection rates are high due to exposure to the causative agent during health care. Likewise, nursing professionals perform their care work maintaining direct contact with patients during working hours of eight hours in general. Therefore, it is evident that there is a high risk of infection for nurses and the health care team; however, patient care in any other area also results in a risk of infection due to the existence of asymptomatic cases.The protective measures provided by national and international health organizations, as well as research products, are fundamental for the care of those they care for. For its part, the Pan American Health Organization (PAHO) prepared a document entitled "Recommendations for the Reorganization and Progressive Expansion of Health Services for the Response to the COVID-19 Pandemic", in which it issued recommendations for optimal internal management in the health centers involved; these recommendations have been updated as new scientific evidence regarding SARS-COV-2 and COVID19 becomes available and which generally includes information on:(6)

• Reorganization and strengthening of the first level of care's response capacity.
• Centralized bed management mechanism.
• Protocol for the diagnosis and sampling of patients with suspected COVID-19.
• Separate triage, care and diagnostic testing flows for respiratory symptomatic patients compatible with suspected COVID-19 cases.
• Conversion, habilitation and complexization of beds according to clinical risk and nursing care dependency.
• Strengthening of home care with or without telehealth.

• Coordination with pre-hospital care services network (emergency care and medical transport devices: ambulances).
• Networked clinical management for continuity of care and efficient use of hospital resources.
• Reorganization, recruitment and training of personnel with emphasis on security and personal protection.
• Strengthened supply chain.

In the same sense, the WHO made technical recommendations required for the protection of occupational health in which it is indicated that after contact with a suspected or confirmed patient it is required to adopt standard precautions, contact and airborne, which are found in the Mexican Official Standard NOM- 045-SSA2-2005, For epidemiological surveillance, prevention and control of nosocomial infections(7) (8).

Within the framework of the above considerations, the research and scientific literature also contains information and protective measures for health personnel during the COVID-19 pandemic; however, all of these are based on the need to evaluate the environment, that is, their recommendations should be adapted according to the context of each country, taking into account the characteristics of the respective health systems.In this regard, Article 4 of the Political Constitution of the United Mexican States ratifies the right to health protection that must be in accordance with certain principles such as equity, universality and free access, which empowers the Ministry of Health to have the obligation to dictate, in case of pandemics, the measures necessary to protect the health of the population. In the first article of the article, it stated: "Avoiding attendance to work centers, public spaces and other crowded places, to elderly adults of 65 years of age or older and groups of people at risk of developing serious illness and/or dying from it, who will enjoy their salary and other benefits established in the current regulations".Based on the above, the nursing professionals who were on the front line in the care of COVID-19 positive patients were working long hours due to the reduction of personnel because of risk factors. In other words, the health team presented an unfavorable panorama of care, where the number of active personnel providing their services was not sufficient for the number of patients requiring care, even though the government hired around 38,583 nursing professionals.(9,10)

Similarly, in Latin America, outpatient consultation rooms and emergency waiting areas tend to be permanently congested and have considerable waiting times, which contributes to the spread of the disease. In addition to coronavirus infection, it coincides with the epidemiological peak of dengue fever, as well as with other contagious diseases prevalent in our environment such as HIV and tuberculosis, making it difficult to concentrate resources and compromising the possibility of carrying out the necessary contingency plans to comply with biosecurity protocols. Likewise, the cost of personal protective equipment means that countries with limited resources will have difficulty in acquiring it, thus leading to the reuse of such equipment that should be discarded after a single use, or to the poor quality of the products, putting the biosafety of health personnel at risk. To summarize the factors that have influenced the predisposition of health personnel to contract the disease while working in health facilities, we can generalize 3 main causes: 1) that emergency personnel did not have training in a new virus, which they had no experience with,This has led to frequent changes in the protocols of care, predisposing to error and confusion; 2) that the disease can manifest itself with mild symptoms, atypical symptoms or even behave asymptomatically, so that health agents exposed infected patients who looked healthy or consulted for other reasons, generating a false sense of security and 3) that due to the high transmissibility of the virus, biosecurity equipment is required which is costly, uncomfortable, and must be disposed of after use, which leads to a lack of resources to adequately address the situation.(11)

Nursing mental health during the COVID 19 pandemic.

Job stress is defined by the WHO as the reaction that an individual may have to work demands and pressures that are not in line with his or her knowledge and abilities and that test his or her ability to cope with the situation. In general, work stress is closely related to the organization of work, the clarification of work activities and the conditions of employment, i.e. psychosocial risks.(12)

It should be noted that the SARS-COV-2 pandemic, as previously mentioned, has put great pressure on health systems and on all health care personnel, such as nurses, who have had to adapt to work in unusual situations, resulting in high levels of stress and emotional burdens.(13)

Consequently, during the pandemic, nurses have found themselves in a situation of panic generated by the fear of contracting the disease and thus transmitting the disease to all those around them, or even transmitting it without being infected, this from a vision in which health caregivers, through the inanimate objects they carry, such as clothing, this is possible because they are the first responders in the line of combat against the pandemic and that has been amplified by several factors.In addition, some situations such as psychological pressure, workload, mediatization, judicial aspects, lack of protection, lack of rest, new roles, discrimination and aggressions of any kind are some of the circumstances that health professionals have been facing, being not only internal but also external conditions that may have an influence on health, performance, job satisfaction and personal satisfaction (14).

On the other hand, other professions not linked to health care and that, depending on their nature, were taken remotely, in addition to having the possibility of having an excused absence that favored a certain population group, however, the nursing personnel able to continue working could not for reasons inherent to the profession, where they were even those who put their lives at risk in the performance of their duties.Naturally, the organism is prepared to face stressful situations; however, this capacity is determined by the characteristics of the stressful stimulus, the characteristics of the receiver, its strategies and coping resources. Considering the above, the balance is not favored towards those workers because the working conditions have not been the necessary to face a health crisis of such magnitude and when the person is unable to fully adapt to factors perceived as threatening or to an excessive demand, distress develops, this is an emotional discomfort of physical, psychological, social and spiritual nature that can interfere with the ability to cope with stressful situations such as those that have been the daily life of health personnel.Due to the above, it is important to recognize distress, as it has a negative impact on the professionals themselves, the patients and the organization of the health team, being also a route to professional burnout and burnout, which is characterized by compassion fatigue, depression, emotional distancing, increased errors in patient care and decreased job satisfaction, which can cause staff to be at risk of developing mood disorders, anxiety and substance abuse, a decrease in the quality of clinical care of patients and consequently increasing the risk of making errors in medical care and a decrease in the degree of patient satisfaction with the care received by health systems. (14)

Therefore, it is relevant to pay due attention to health personnel in a comprehensive manner, through public policies that allow both individual and organizational strategies and leadership styles and more research to establish which interventions are more effective in specific populations and how individual and organizational

solutions can be combined to obtain better results and prevent caregivers from becoming patients who, instead of providing, require medical care. (15)
Perception of the work context of nursing personnel.

It has been shown that throughout the pandemic there was an increase in the prevalence of anxiety and depression diagnoses. These are exacerbated by work stress, work overload, isolation, and discrimination, aspects that are related to the care of people with SARS-COV-2.In other words, during the pandemic there were cases of physical and verbal aggression to health personnel in the public area, this discrimination negatively affected the perspective of the staff, decreasing the mood, social interaction, adding to this the aggression that was received by social networks increased the stigmatization and violence towards health personnel, Many opted to change their clothes and not to wear their uniforms outside the work area to avoid being a target of aggressions, since in addition to the overloaded environment that was experienced inside the hospital, social rejection was occasionally added in the public thoroughfare.It should be noted that there was also an increase in diagnoses of anxiety and depression in the personnel, considering within this the fear of the risk of contagion that existed among the health personnel and their families, whose cause of stress was the most frequent, as well as the fact that all those health professionals of younger age and minimal work experience are affected by these ailments, unlike experienced personnel who dominate the environment and have a greater capacity for resilience in an emergency situation. It has been identified that the lack of The lack of family support coupled with the isolation of health care workers to prevent infection has had repercussions on health care workers as part of the stress and fear during the pandemic.Consequently. Nurses who have also been directly involved with patients in intensive care during the COVID 19 pandemic, with high exposure to the risk of infection and even increased workload, have reported fear, uncertainty, nervousness and anxiety about contracting the disease and infecting people in their close environment, They also feel anguish and a sense of guilt for not being able to provide optimal care to their own family members, and the work overload has affected their physical health through insomnia, recurrent headaches, anxiety crises, panic attacks, and difficulty breathing, which directly affects their work performance. Although, in another sense, the lack of research and truthfulness about the disease was not an impediment to fulfill the corresponding tasks, since the personnel kept carrying out their activities in spite of being uncertain about the disease, waiting for the results of research that would provide more information about the virus, later they had to face the excess of information and false information that was dispersed among the population. The nursing staff found it necessary to exercise a leadership role in order to manage the organization and comply with the requirements of providing good patient care. The saturation of hospitals during the COVID 19 pandemic has shown us that human resources and the reorganization of activities through good management is what has been the basis for patient care, given the specificity of the care required by patients and despite the transfer of specialist nurses, it was necessary to request the support of new staff to provide sufficient supply for patient care (16,17).

Conclusion

Health professionals have been a pillar during this pandemic, at the forefront of community care, offering solutions, being able to reinvent the health system to respond to this social and health emergency, nurses in various fields of action such as health centers, nursing homes and hospitals have led the implementation of all processes and circuits with generosity and absolute dedication, each professional has contributed to innovate in their day to day, while fulfilling their principles in order to provide holistic care to each person, and in the same way including not only the patient, but also their relatives who from another perspective also require support from the nursing staff, due to the process of anguish and concern associated with their families who go through this condition, despite the constant changes of protocols, all staff has been responsible for managing the changes in all units, making easy the difficult, and once again, being next to the people who need our care, our support, and our accompaniment to the final farewell.On the other hand, it is important to mention that this long period has brought with it significant lessons, that teamwork has been streamlined and evidenced both inside and outside the hospital area, it has allowed the use of new means of communication, the improvement of many projects, and it has also been demonstrated worldwide how important it is to take care of integral health from home,At present, health personnel are still alert to all requirements, certain safety protocols continue to be followed for the good of the population, although the use of protective equipment has worked correctly, there are still areas of opportunity with respect to occupational health in the hospital area, likewise, it is necessary to delve a little deeper into the mental health of both professionals and the population in general, since this event has left a historical mark and as a means of protection, this important point should be prioritized, in order to improve the quality of life of the individual.

References

1. Ferrer R. COVID-19 pandemic: the greatest challenge in the history of intensive care. Med Intensiva [Internet]. August 1, 2020 [cited June 17, 2022];44(6):323-4. Available at: http://www.medintensiva.org/es-pandemia-por-covid-19-el-mayor-articulo-S0210569120301017

2. Health S de. COVID-19 FREQUENTLY ASKED QUESTIONS [Internet]. gob.mx. [cited 2022 June 17]. Available from: http://www.gob.mx/salud/documentos/covid-19-preguntas-frecuentes?state=published

3. Maguiña Vargas C, Gastelo Acosta R, Tequen Bernilla A, Maguiña Vargas C, Gastelo Acosta R, Tequen Bernilla A. The new Coronavirus and the Covid-19 pandemic. Rev Medica Hered [Internet]. April 2020 [cited June 17, 2022];31(2):125-31. Available from: http://www.scielo.org.pe/scielo.php?script=sci_abstract&pid=S1018-130X2020000200125&lng=en&nrm=iso&tlng=en.

4. Loyola da Silva TC, de Medeiros Pinheiro Fernandes ÁK, Brito do O'Silva C, de Mesquita Xavier SS, Bezerra de Macedo EA, Loyola da Silva TC, et al. The impact of the pandemic on the role of nursing: a narrative review of the literature. Enferm Glob [Internet]. 2021 [cited 2022 Jun 17];20(63):502-43. Available from: https://scielo.isciii.es/scielo.php?script=sci_abstract&pid=S1695-61412021210003000016&lng=en&nrm=iso&tlng=en.

5. Cadena-Estrada JC, Olvera-Arreola SS, López-Flores L, Pérez-Hernández E, Lira-Rodríguez G, Sánchez-Cisneros N, et al. Nursing in the face of COVID-19, a key point for the prevention, control and mitigation of the pandemic. Arch Cardiol México [Internet]. 2020 [cited 2022 June 17];90:94-9. Available from: http://www.scielo.org.mx/scielo.php?script=sci_abstract&pid=S1405-99402020000500094&lng=en&nrm=iso&tlng=en

6. OPSHSSHSCOVID-19200018_spa.pdf [Internet]. [cited 2022 June 17]. Available from: https://iris.paho.org/bitstream/handle/10665.2/52214/OPSHSSHSCOVID-19200018_spa.pdf?sequence=1&isAllowed=y

7. WHO-2019-nCoV-IHR-Quarantine-2021.1-spa.pdf [Internet]. [cited 2022 Jun 29, 2022]. Available from: https://apps.who.int/iris/bitstream/handle/10665/342649/WHO-2019-nCoV-IHR-Quarantine-2021.1-spa.pdf.

8. DOF - Official Journal of the Federation [Internet]. [cited 29 June 2022]. Available from: https://dof.gob.mx/nota_detalle.php?codigo=5120943&fecha=20/11/2009

9. 004. Continuity of employment for nurses who joined the fight against COVID-19: Insabi | Secretaría de Salud | Gobierno | gob.mx [Internet]. [cited 17 June 2022]. Available from: https://www.gob.mx/salud/prensa/004-continuidad- laboral-al-personal-de-enfermeria-que-se-sumo-a-la-lucha-contra-covid-19- insabi?idiom=en.

10. Morales Aguirre AM, Choy Gómez J, Mariñelarena Mariñelarena JL, López Gavito E. The legal vision in Mexico of the COVID-19 contingency. Cir Gen [Internet]. 2020 [cited 2022 June 17];42(2):109-15. Available from: https://www.medigraphic.com/cgi-bin/new/resumen.cgi?IDARTICULO=95369

11. Valdés PR, Cámera LA, Serna M de la, Abuabara-Turbay Y, Carballo-Zárate V, Hernández-Ayazo H, et al. Attack on health care personnel during the COVID-19 pandemic in Latin America. Acta Medica Colomb [Internet]. September 2020 [cited June 17, 2022];45(3):55-69. Available at: http://www.scielo.org.co/scielo.php?script=sci_abstract&pid=S0120-24482020000300055&lng=pt&nrm=iso&tlng=en

12. Mitchell C, https://www.facebook.com/pahowho. PAHO/WHO | Job stress is a burden on individuals, workers, and societies [Internet]. Pan American Health Organization / World Health Organization. 2016 [cited 2016 Jun 17, 2022]. Available from:

13. https://www3.paho.org/hq/index.php?option=com_content&view=article&id=11973: work place-stress-takes-a-toll-on-individuals-employers-and-

societies&Itemid=135&lang=en.

14. Peiró T, Lorente L, Vera M. The COVID-19 Crisis: Skills That Are Paramount to Build into Nursing Programs for Future Global Health Crisis. Int J Environ Res Public Health [Internet]. January 2020 [cited June 17, 2022];17(18):6532. Available from: https://www.mdpi.com/1660-4601/17/18/6532

15. Moral distress and burnout in health care personnel during covid-19 crisis - ScienceDirect [Internet]. [cited 2022 Jun 17, 2022]. Available from: https://www.sciencedirect.com/science/article/pii/S0716864020301000

16. García-Iglesias JJ, Gómez-Salgado J, Martín-Pereira J, Fagundo-Rivera J, Ayuso-Murillo D, Martínez-Riera JR. Impact of sars-cov-2 (covid-19) on the mental health of health professionals: a systematic review. Rev Esp Public Health. :20.

17. Wauters M, Zamboni Berra T, de Almeida Crispim J, Arcêncio RA, Cartagena-Ramos D. Quality of life of health personnel during the COVID-19 pandemic: exploratory review. Rev Panam Salud Publica [Internet]. May 2, 2022 [cited 2022 Jun 17];46:e30. Available from: https://www.ncbi.nlm.nih.gov/pmc/articles/PMC9060205/

18. González-Gil MT, Oter-Quintana C, Martínez-Marcos M, Alcolea-Cosín MT, Navarta-Sánchez MV, Robledo-Martín J, et al. The value of human resources: Experience of critical care nurses during the COVID-19 epidemic. Enferm Intensiva [Internet]. 2022 [cited 2022 Jun 17];33(2):77-88. Available from: https://www.ncbi.nlm.nih.gov/pmc/articles/PMC9068597/

CHAPTER 7

ETHICAL AND LEGAL FRAMEWORK IN OCCUPATIONAL HEALTH

Janet Carolina Negrón Espadas ** Aurora Sierra Canto ***
José Fernando Loria Polanco * Diego Manuel Martín Chan * Diego Manuel Martín Chan * José Fernando Loria Polanco * Diego Manuel Martín Chan * Diego Manuel Martín Chan

After so many years studying ethics, I have come to the conclusion that it can be summed up in three virtues: courage to live, generosity to live together, and prudence to survive.

Fernando Savater, 1947.

Introduction

The following chapter presents the legal ethical aspects that contribute to the practice of occupational health that protect the health of workers and promote the establishment and maintenance of a safe and healthy work environment, as well as encourage the adaptation of work to the capabilities of workers, in favor of their health that facilitate preventive work aimed at providing a safe and healthy work environment for all, under the premise of three concepts that allow the achievement of the above mentioned: basic principles, obligations and rights of workers in health. The method used was a bibliographic review of legal documents and updated scientific articles.At the outset, it is important to mention that the discipline of occupational health ethics has developed rapidly in recent decades. Focusing primarily on articulating and exploring the ethical issues that arise in the pursuit of the health of women and men in the workplace.

*Student of the Bachelor's Degree in Nursing. Autonomous University of Yucatan

workers. This has led to an emphasis on concepts such as the common good, equity, solidarity, reciprocity and welfare without neglecting important ethical considerations and more individual values such as autonomy and privacy.

In recent years there has been an increased interest at the international, regional and national levels in the protection of workers' health and safety and the environmental conditions in which they work.In this regard, the figures presented by the International Labor Organization (ILO, 2016) reveal that approximately 2.78 million people die due to accidents and diseases related to work, and that more than 374 million accidents are reported each year. The ILO mentions that for companies they represent a large increase in costs, of which these can reach 4% of the global Gross Domestic Product (GDP), and that these are mostly produced by poor safety and health practices. In a decent job there is freedom for workers to express their opinions and participate in labor decisions that affect their lives in equal opportunity, personal development, business competitiveness (Tomasina, 2012), in a framework of safety and labor protection.In 2007, the WHO stated that half of the world's population is made up of workers, who are the main generators of economic and social development and growth. Of this population, only a small minority has access to occupational health services (OHS) and they are related to: primary prevention of occupational hazards; health promotion; working conditions and improvement of workers' health programs and systems, coinciding with the three objectives promulgated by the Code of Ethics of the International Commission on Occupational Health (ICOH).We are currently experiencing a new paradigm for occupational health, which although it contemplates the classic focus on "health risk management" also includes medical aspects in health, acquiring greater importance in recent years in the prevention of hazards and the promotion of health. Thus, nowadays, occupational health The ethical aspects of health protection, as well as the promotion of health in the workplace, must be taken into account.

Work ethics in the modern world

In the last decade, codes of ethics have been approved for the various branches of medicine and occupational health professionals at the international and national levels. Therefore, it is necessary to recognize their responsibilities, even though they can be classified as complicated and even conflicting.The importance of ethics in this area lies primarily in the responsibilities of those involved in the company, such as occupational health professionals, administrative personnel, authorities, judicial and social security bodies.Second, the recent increase in the number of poorly trained occupational health professionals, including those in charge of occupational safety, due to institutional needs to create mandatory or voluntary positions to provide occupational health services.In addition to these two reasons, another element to consider is the importance of developing an interdisciplinary, multisectoral and specialized approach.In other words, occupational health professionals are those persons who carry out activities in the field of occupational health and safety at work, who provide services or who are part of the practice of occupational health, under the codes of ethics in force.

Basic principles

The purpose of occupational health is to serve the health and social welfare of workers individually and collectively. The practice of occupational health should be conducted in accordance with the highest professional standards and rigorous ethical principles.Occupational health professionals have different obligations that include the protection of the life and health of workers, respect for human dignity, the promotion of ethical principles in health policies and programs, and the promotion of the health and safety of workers. occupational. They must also have integrity in professional conduct, impartiality and protection of the confidentiality of workers' health data and privacy. These professionals must be experts with the capacity for professional independence in the exercise of their functions, as well as acquire the necessary competence to fulfill their obligations and demand the conditions that will allow them to carry out their activities in accordance with good practice and professional ethics.On the other hand, health personnel have a series of rights and obligations that, if violated and/or not complied with, lead to lawsuits and their respective substantiation before the various competent authorities, in these cases to criminal, civil and administrative judicial actions that will elucidate the respective liability.

Duties and obligations of occupational health professionals

Objectives and advisory role. The purpose of the occupational health practice is to preserve and promote the health of workers as a result of a healthy and safe working environment, as well as to protect the working capacity of workers and their access to employment. To achieve these objectives, valid risk assessment methods must be used, effective preventive measures must be proposed and their implementation must be monitored. However, occupational health professionals should provide honest advice to employers on how to fulfill their occupational health and safety responsibilities.

Knowledge and experience. Occupational health professionals should strive to remain familiar with the work and work environment, as well as improve their competence and keep themselves well informed about scientific and technical knowledge, occupational hazards and the most efficient ways to eliminate or reduce risks.

Development of a policy and program. It should be emphasized that it is essential to advise management and workers on the factors existing in the company that may affect health. Therefore, the evaluation of occupational risks should be directed to the establishment of an occupational health and safety policy and a prevention program adapted to the company's needs. Therefore, such policy and program should be proposed based on the available updated scientific and technical knowledge.

Emphasis on prevention and immediate action. Attention should be given to the rapid application of simple prevention measures that are highly reliable and easy to implement. Subsequently, it should be verified whether the measures adopted are effective or whether more complete solutions are required. When there are doubts about the severity of an occupational hazard, immediate precautionary actions should be taken and assumed as necessary.

Safety and health information. With respect to health and safety information, occupational health professionals should contribute to providing information to workers on the occupational risks to which they are exposed in an objective and understandable manner, without hiding any facts and highlighting preventive measures. They should also cooperate with the employer, workers and their representatives to ensure that they provide adequate occupational health and safety information and training to management and workers.

Health surveillance. Another important aspect to mention is that the objectives, methods and procedures of health surveillance must be clearly defined, giving priority to the adaptation of workplaces to workers, who must receive all the information in this regard. Therefore, this surveillance will be carried out with the informed consent of the workers. For this reason, as part of the process of obtaining consent, workers should be informed about the possible positive or negative consequences resulting from their participation in the implementation of screening and health surveillance programs.

Information to the employer. It should be emphasized that the results of examinations prescribed by national legislation or regulations should only be reported to the company management on fitness for the intended work, or on medically necessary limitations on the assignment of tasks or on exposure to certain occupational hazards, with emphasis on proposals to adapt the tasks and working conditions to the worker's aptitudes.

Dangers to third parties. Another important point is that the employee must be informed when his or her state of health or the nature of the tasks he or she performs at his or her workplace may endanger the safety of third parties. Therefore, in the event of particularly dangerous situations, the management of the company and the competent authority must be informed of the measures necessary to protect others.

Health promotion. One of the most important components is health promotion; therefore, employers and workers should be encouraged to participate in the design and implementation of health education, health promotion, health risk detection and public health programs. They should take measures to ensure the confidentiality of workers' personal health data, and should prevent its misuse.

Workers' rights

Regarding the rights of workers it should be said that when talking about carrying out the work of professions, their main and complementary activities involving human resources, it is regularized by the following laws:

• The Regulatory Law of Article 5 of the Mexican Constitution, which relates to the practice of professions at the federal level, published in the Official Gazette of the Federation of May 26, 1945, first section (Ley de Profesiones).

• Coordination bases that are currently in accordance with the law and are defined by the educational and health authorities.

• The guidelines of the General Health Law

• Laws issued by the states, based on articles 5° and 121, section V, of the Federal Constitution.

Rights in the exercise of the profession.

Article 5 of the Federal Constitution establishes that health personnel have the right to the following:

• Health professionals, as part of their obligation to assist the health of dam workers, should have the right to request, if necessary, additional examinations to those established as a minimum requirement by national regulatory laws.

• In addition, to exercise their profession freely, as long as it is within the framework of legality,

• Undoubtedly, not to be deprived of the freedom to practice their profession in their personal way of the professional, except when the judicial area determines it, and when the rights of third parties are violated, or by governmental decision, according to the terms established by law, when the rights of society are violated.

• However, in the case of social service or professional services of a social nature, the remuneration shall be obtained in accordance with the provisions of the law, with the respective exceptions indicated therein.

• Likewise, no contract, pact or agreement shall be entered into with the purpose of detracting from the loss or irrevocable sacrifice of its own freedom for any reason whatsoever.

• Lastly, do not enter into any agreement whereby you temporarily or permanently renounce the exercise of your profession.

Labor rights

• With respect to Article 5 of the Political Constitution of the United Mexican States, the rights are as follows:

• Fair remuneration for rendering their personal labor and their full consent, except in the case of work imposed as a penalty by the judicial authority, which shall be determined as imposed in fractions I and II of Article 123.

• Not to be deprived of the fruits of one's labor, only by judicial resolution.
• That the labor contract only obliges him/her to render the agreed service for the time established by law, without the capacity to exceed one year to the detriment of the

The employee's right to work, and cannot be extended in any case, to the renouncement, loss or distortion of any political or civil rights.

• In the case of the fulfillment of such contract, as far as the employee is concerned, he/she may only be obliged to the corresponding civil liability, and in no case may his/her person be coerced.

Pursuant to article 123 of the Constitution, it will be concluded that one has the right to:
• To have a dignified and socially useful job.

Specific rights of health personnel

Now, in accordance with the General Health Law, the following rights are identified:
To enjoy the necessary training for human resources, which will meet the standards and criteria issued by the educational authorities, in coordination with the health authorities, with the participation of higher education institutions (Article 79).Conscientious objection, in the Federal District, a physician who is required to perform a legal termination of pregnancy and whose religious beliefs or personal convictions are contrary to such procedure, may be a conscientious objector and for that reason may excuse himself/herself from performing the termination of pregnancy, having the obligation to refer the woman to a physician who is not a conscientious objector. When the legal termination of pregnancy is urgent to safeguard the health or life of the woman, conscientious objection may not be invoked (Article 59 of the General Health Law of the Federal District).Enjoy the training and updating provided by the health authorities, without prejudice to the competence that corresponds to the educational authorities and in coordination with them, as well as with the participation of educational institutions (Article 89).Voluntary participation of health professionals, technicians and auxiliaries in teaching activities (Article 90).

Conclusions

For nurses, ethics is a guide for decision making when providing care, to ensure the adherence of their actions to the values and duties of the profession.In view of this fact, it is necessary to bear in mind that the approach to occupational health is multidisciplinary. Since, there is a wide range of obligations, duties, rights and complex relationships between people working in this field. It is therefore important to define the roles of each of the occupational health professionals with other professionals, and with their peers in the field of development, economic, social and health policies. This work requires a clear vision of the ethics of occupational health professionals and the standards of their professional conduct.It is also important to emphasize the importance of good professional ethics on the part of occupational health professionals for the development of an adequate environment for workers, in addition to knowledge regarding the rights and obligations that belong to each member of the team for the correct development of their work competencies, as well as each of the laws that are responsible for protecting workers.

References

• Delgado-Arteaga LJ, Borroto-Cruz ER, Moreira-Macías EL. Occupational safety and health regulations and ethical issues. Revista San Gregorio [Internet]. 2020 [cited June 17, 2022];(40):176-200. Available from: http://scielo.senescyt.gob.ec/scielo.php?script=sci_arttext&pid=S2528-79072020000300176

• Code of ethics for occupational health professionals, December 1991 [Internet]. Latin American Journal of Occupational Health; 2001. [cited 2022 June 17]; Available from: https://www.medigraphic.com/pdfs/trabajo/lm-2001/lm012b.pdf.

• International Code of Ethics for Occupational Health Professionals [Internet]. [cited 2022 Jun 17, 2022]; Available from: https://higieneyseguridadlaboralcvs.files.wordpress.com/2012/08/codigo_etico.pd f

• Lavicoli, A., Valenti, A., Gagliardi, D., Rantanen, J. Ethics and occupational health in the contemporary world. [Internet]. Environ. Res. Public Health; 2018. [cited 2022 Jun 17, 2022]; Available from: https://smiba.org.ar/curso_medico_especialista/lecturas_2021/%C3%89tica%20y%20salud%20ocupacional%20en%20el%20mundo%20laboral%20contempor%C3%A1neo.pdf

• ILO. Technical and ethical guiding principles concerning workers' health surveillance. [Internet]. Geneva, International Labour Office, 1998. [cited 17 June 2022]; Available from: https://www.ilo.org/wcmsp5/groups/public/@dgreports/@dcomm/@publ/documents/publication/wcms_publ_9223108284_en.pdf.

• Hernández, M. Rights of health personnel. [Internet]. Mexico City. : Instituto Nacional de Estudios Históricos de las Revoluciones de México, Universidad Nacional Autónoma de México, Instituto de Investigaciones Jurídicas, 2015; 73 pages. [cited 2022 June 17]; Available from: https://www.inehrm.gob.mx/work/models/Constitucion1917/Resource/1412/PDF_Derechos_del_personal_de_salud.pdf.

• Pan American Health Organization. Plan of Action on Workers' Health. [internet]. Washington; 2015. [cited 2015 June 17, 2022]. Available from: http://www.paho.org/hq/index.php?option=com_docman&task=doc_download&gid=31677&Itemid=270&lang=en.

Arenas, Á., Riveros, C. Ethical and legal aspects of occupational health. [internet]. Pers.bioét. 2017;21(1): 62-77. [cited 2022 Jun 17, 2022]. Available from: https://www.redalyc.org/pdf/832/83250156005.pdf

CHAPTER 8

PSYCHOSOCIAL RISK FACTORS IN HEALTH PROFESSIONALS.

Aurora sierra canto** Alejandra Liset Toloza May* Alejandra Saraí Kantún Pech* Alejandra Saraí Kantún Pech* Alejandra Liset Toloza May* Alejandra Saraí Kantún Pech

Security is not expensive, it is invaluable.

Jerry Smith

Introduction

Nowadays, globalization and other factors such as competitiveness in the work environment, as well as the increase in the hiring of workers, productivity and even insecurity in the work area, are elements that cause precariousness and deterioration in the adequate conditions that health personnel need for the correct performance of their duties.(1)It is imperative to consider that psychosocial risk factors are present in the work area of health professionals, and affect different dimensions, which can range from the most common ones such as psychological, to personal or autonomous issues.In this regard, the International Labor Organization (ILO) defines psychosocial factors as: "The interactions between the content, organization and management of work and environmental conditions, on the one hand, and the functions and needs of workers, on the other. These interactions could exert a harmful influence on the health of workers through their perceptions and experience."(1)

*Student of the Bachelor's Degree in Nursing. Autonomous University of Yucatan

**Career Professor. Faculty of Nursing. Autonomous University of Yucatan

Psychosocial risk factors are derived from and depend on the functions of the worker, their environment and long working hours with a high workload, as these cause various disorders such as increased stress and anxiety due to poor adaptation. They are those inadequate conditions that cause distemper in the health of workers, these in turn cause occupational diseases of different types that externalize the working conditions in which workers are, reducing the functional capacity of the professional to perform at an optimal level.Therefore, scrutinizing risk factors for the benefit of workers has become a subject of extensive study at present, some research on the subject has shown that they are the greatest source of damage to health, welfare and productivity in institutions that are responsible for providing health services. Their detection and intervention would give access to a state of favorable conditions for the worker, i.e., health professionals are considered human resources that constitute the largest workforce, consequently, their absence generates deficits in the care they provide.(2)For some years the absence of any physical illness is no longer considered as a sign of quality health, as shown by the definition of the concept of "Health" according to the World Health Organization (WHO), so it is mentioned the importance of the relationship between physical, mental and social circumstances, so that the work must maintain facilities to ensure welfare conditions for the safety of such workers. Mental health is more than just the absence of mental disorders, since it requires the adaptation of the individual to the context or situation in which he/she may be present, which will determine his/her psychological well-being, despite his/her economic, environmental and social circumstances in the work environment.All in all, the psychosocial risk factors currently present play an important role with respect to mental health vulnerability that are present in healthcare workers in any work setting.(3)

Classification of psychosocial risk factors

The psychosocial risk factors in question are not a new issue in working life, in fact they have been masked and hidden by other factors that have been prioritized, such as ergonomic, physical, chemical and biological risks. It is time for psychosocial risk factors to take center stage because their importance is rooted in today's working conditions.In this chapter, the classification of the four risk factors in health professionals will be appended:

1) Quantitative requirements

They are defined as the amount of work and the time to perform it. The health professional has a wide range of activities ranging from care, education and support, as well as administrative, scientific or research activities, because if anything is certain is that all those who work in the professional area of health require constant updating. All this must be done in a given period of time, performing up to two or more activities simultaneously, exposing them to a high mental workload.The factor associated with exposure to relevant quantitative demands, such as the type of service in which the care is being provided, should also be considered. It is appropriate to highlight the fact that the demands and risk factors are not comparable when the health professional works only in a private office or privately, when he/she works in a health institution, and even more so when the institution where he/she works (whether public or private) provides more specialized care, such as emergency rooms, resuscitation rooms, intensive care units, delivery rooms and oncology services; as these services are known to present greater overload, increased work pace and greater physical and mental exhaustion.(1)Therefore, quantitative demands increase the workload and stress on health care professionals, which sometimes makes them susceptible to perform their activities inefficiently, in addition to the fact that occasionally health care professionals are not able to perform their activities efficiently. activities performed in their role as caregivers, whether personal or in collaborative activities, are undervalued, causing the loss of the essence of a humanized and quality care, failing to see the patient as a holistic being in their care, an issue that should prevail both in the health professional and in the institutions providing services(4).

2) Pace of work

The working conditions or circumstances triggered by changes in the models of contracting, production and provision of services have generated that the health professional is imposed a pace and a strenuous workload, and following this, the institutions seek, for the most part, quantity rather than quality; this means that care is provided to a greater number of patients, with various functions, role activities and attached activities (which are not of the role according to each health professional) in order to increase productivity and "efficiency" to the satisfaction and benefit of the institutions.The pace of work relates production to execution times or deadlines, it is directly related to the standard time, known from the execution of such activities. It is intensified by several factors, among them, the care in services, which due to their complexity, demand greater attention to patients, the lack of personnel in the institutions to cover the demands of care, the double labor linkage and the institutional pressure to increase productivity, to avoid making mistakes and to fulfill the work.The repercussions of overload and high work pace are reflected in the various difficulties in the adaptation processes, reflected in physical and/or mental exhaustion, which can range from a partial or total loss of bodily and/or psychic capacities for the development of daily life activities. It has been demonstrated that an excess of work intensifies stress, as well as the presence of greater psychosomatic symptomatology, expressed in: loss of sleep, alteration of appetite, tiredness, headache and irritability, gastrointestinal changes, immunosuppression, need to use anxiolytics or other medications, decrease or increase of body weight, crying episodes, feeling of sadness, headaches, joint pains and others. Also social, family and professional dynamics can be negatively affected by the lack of time available to share with family and friends in daily life, and time for rest, recreation and professional training is reduced. Due to the amount of stressors that health professionals have to face, they are part of a group highly affected by Burnout syndrome with high levels of burnout.(1)

According to the dictionary of medical terms of the Royal National Academy of Medicine of Spain, Burnout is a syndrome of professional burnout, emotional overload syndrome, burnout syndrome or fatigue syndrome at work was declared, in 2000 by the WHO, as an occupational risk factor, due to its ability to affect the quality of life, mental health and even to put at risk the life of the individual who suffers it. It is described as an inadequate way of coping with chronic stress, the main features of which are emotional exhaustion, depersonalization and decreased personal performance.(5) (6)

3) Double presence

It is related to the simultaneous requirement of people with a personal role at home and a professional role at work (this role is sometimes exacerbated by the requirement to perform work not only in one institution, whether public or private, but in two or more occupations where they are required to perform tasks related to their profession).It is worth highlighting the very marked difference occasionally for the female sex, since historically the patriarchal construct that has accompanied women since the beginning of humanity assigns them the function of care and attention to the basic needs of others in the home, that is, the domestic sphere, where the management of activities involves the care and raising of children, the maintenance of the home and the role with their partner, this only as part of their personal role, increased when there is the existence of a professional role, regardless of their career in the field as a health professional. Dual presence is a stressful factor for health professionals, especially when their work is characterized by shift work, with long and exhausting shifts that force them to work at a faster pace, increasing the emotional and physical demands that can negatively affect both work performance and professional and personal life. In the work environment, the increased physical and psychological load can alter the state of health, affect relationships between colleagues and suffer or commit accidents or work-related errors. In the personal sphere, the repercussions are usually extra-occupational, such as a decrease in family and social contact, reduction of support networks and of leisure activities, thus causing alterations in the state of physical, emotional and mental health and the effects of the non-dissociation of personal and professional life.The repercussions of the double presence can be manifested equally in the difficulty to make decisions, the possibility of making mistakes and the occurrence of accidents inside or outside the home, by moments of drowsiness, tiredness and exhaustion, and alterations of the circadian rhythm (causing alterations in the pattern of sleep and rest)(1). All of this leads to a decrease in professional and personal growth due to the fact that possible present opportunities for training and education that may exist are missed, either due to lack of time, the demands of roles for the performance of activities and even gender inequalities, which would only create a vicious circle of frustration, dissatisfaction and stress.

4) Emotional demands

Emotional demands are the requirements to hide emotions and control expressions of feelings, both positive and negative, in the face of the diversity of circumstances experienced as health professionals, to ensure the correct performance of activities for the patient and the fulfillment of the work as part of the satisfaction requirements of the institution.The exposure of health care professionals to this psychosocial risk factor in the hospital area is astounding, since they are constantly exposed to this risk factor in the work environment.The demands of care by the patient, family members and colleagues of the health and administrative team in their multidisciplinary functions also have an impact.These demands occur when faced with complex situations, mainly in mental health, emergency and intensive care services, in which they interact with critically ill, conflictive, dying or especially complex individuals. The coexistence with human suffering and death is perhaps the most stressful factor, as well as the confrontation in making difficult decisions, from which ethical and moral implications are frequently derived.(1) These situations generate both work stress and physical, mental and emotional exhaustion; one must consider the exponential sum of situations that in the personal role may aggravate these demands, exposing the professional to emotions of suffering, pain, hopelessness, worry, fear, disconsolation, helplessness and anguish.For its part, the National Institute of Safety and Hygiene at Work groups psychosocial risk factors into: 1) Tasks. These are the required characteristics related to the performance of the work activity, such as work rhythm, role conflict and ambiguity, monotony and repetitiveness of the task, autonomy, mental workload, qualification and professional status; 2) Organization of work time. This refers to the organization and content of work in terms of time; it involves issues such as working hours, shift work and night work; and 3) Structure of work organization. This refers to all the necessary aspects that are required to obtain the product or the performance of the work, i.e., the expected end result of the various work activities; such as formal organization, work processes, rules, human resources practices and internal culture.According to the ILO, these psychosocial risk factors represent a set of perceptions and experiences of the worker that include: 1) Individual or personal factors of the worker, which can include illnesses as well as emotional or mental states of the worker that are part of his daily personal life; 2) The working conditions and environment, which refer to all those related to stressors in the work area, which can be work conditions (such as the work environment, infrastructure, preventive measures, tasks and organizational factors) and workers' reactions (depending on their skills, needs, expectations, culture and private life) and 3) External factors, which include economic and social conditions outside the workplace that have an impact on it.

Impact, identification and analysis of psychosocial risk factors.

The impact of psychosocial risk factors, according to Moreno and Báez, generally classifies them into three levels: 1) At the first level, they generate positive, negative and adaptive responses; 2) At the second level, they generate harmful effects on workers' health and organizational functioning; and 3) At the third level, these psychosocial risks have a high probability of affecting workers' health and business functioning in the medium and long term.Naturally, performing job functions and achieving the desired results for any job can cause workers to develop stressors that can lead to conditions that affect their behavior, mood and organ status, including physical illness, as mentioned above. Over the years, due importance has been given to the impact these factors have on quality of life as a consequence of such jobs where the workload and responsibilities are constantly increasing.(7)Once the risks are classified, the probability and severity of their consequences are critical. Among the most common psychosocial risks, generally speaking, we can find Burnout syndrome, workaholism, technical stress, ergo dependency, ADHD, as well as people may find themselves dealing with anxiety and fatigue due to work overload. For its part, the Mexican Institute of Social Security (IMSS) identifies the main psychosocial risks, most of them previously mentioned, that occur in Mexico: work stress, violence at work, workplace harassment, sexual harassment, insecurity, Burnout syndrome, conflicts that exist in relation to work-family and emotional work. These come to cause disorders or certain affectations, which are attributed to the workload that is distributed inadequately, since it can manifest a failure in terms of leadership, causing it to be of a negative nature, although these consequences that are manifested in the welfare of people, are reported by three out of four workers (8).

Over the years, the WHO, the IMSS and the National Autonomous University of Mexico (UNAM) have identified mental and behavioral disorders that have a significant impact on health, economic and labor issues. For example, it is estimated that 25% of patients who use the health system do so because of a mental disorder, and it is also predicted that by 2025 mental disorders will be the main cause of occupational disability, thanks to which the Ministry of Labor and Social Welfare determines that psychosocial risk is responsible for 50 to 60% of lost work hours.(9)

On the other hand, the identification and analysis of risk factors should contemplate the following: 1) Conditions in the work environment. This refers to the fact that the work environment should not be dangerous, unsafe, deficient or unhealthy, requiring an additional effort to adapt to the work environment. 2) Workloads. Refers to the imposition of work for the employee that exceeds his or her capacity. 3) Lack of control over the work. It is the little or no possibility that the employee has to influence and make decisions in the performance of their activities, contrary to the initiative and autonomy for the use and development of skills and knowledge. 4) Working hours and shift rotation that exceed the provisions of the Federal Labor Law. The working time in terms, duration and schedule are extensive, without regular breaks and rests, nor preventive and protective measures to diagnose any health condition. 5) Interference in the work-family relationship. This is when there is a conflict between family or personal activities and work duties. 6) Negative leadership and negative relationships at work. These are the characteristics and qualities of the employer or his representatives that are aggressive, imposing or negative and have a direct influence on the performance of workers. 7) Conforming labor violence, being those acts of physical, emotional and psychological harassment, bullying and mistreatment.

Workers' rights

Having the right to work is fundamental and essential for other human rights to become known, as it includes a part that cannot be separated from human dignity, since it is considered that in order for every person to live with dignity, he/she must have the right to work. When considering the right to work, three important elements are taken into account(10):1) Freedom to be able to perform a lawful job without the intervention of any public authority. 2) To take into account that the realization of a job entails positive obligations to promote and generate new jobs. 3) The work should be carried out under fair conditionsIt is considered that this represents an important impact in the economic, political and social spheres, which is why it is considered a necessity and is only carried out in a meticulous manner, since enforcing these labor rights ensures that people who have a job where they enjoy these benefits are provided and can exercise them in a dignified and correct manner, in conditions of equality in salary, gender and without any type of discrimination.(11) It is important to take into account two spheres that are handled in the work environment, the individual and the collective; although the work environment involves certain aspects that, as mentioned above, affect the quality of life and even the physical integrity of employees, violating to a certain degree the rights they obtain at work. Firstly, we are going to refer to the conditions that a person must meet to fully develop at work, for example, to be trained, to be free from exploitation, to feel safe in a hygienic work environment and therefore with a reasonable work schedule, to be able to enjoy vacations, to be able to remain or be promoted at work, without exclusion or dismissal in any discriminatory way. With respect to the collective sphere, issues related to the formation and/or free and independent integration of trade unions or associations for the defense of their rights and the improvement of their working conditions are covered. workers named as "Strike" to enforce the rights they are being deprived of.(12,13)

In Mexico, the rights of workers are found in Articles 5 and 123 of the Political Constitution of the United Mexican States, as well as the regulatory laws of the Federal Labor Law and the Federal Law of Workers in the Service of the State, which protect and protect the right to work, as well as the right to obtain an adequate income, referring to the fact that a person works for what he/she should receive a remuneration that allows him/her to have a dignified life.Human rights focused on the labor area also include the right to have social security by the workplace, to have access to health systems and to have protection through the institutions in charge of providing them, and to make use of these services in case of illness, accidents, either in general or in the work environment, Similarly, if there is any occupational hazard, widowhood or orphanhood, pensions for incapacity for work, which become part of a minimum of this corresponding social security that such employers are required to provide to their workers, since they are considered as human rights that describe a decent and adequate job.(14)

The Political Constitution of the United Mexican States, as previously mentioned, states in Article 123 that "Every person has the right to dignified and socially useful work", indicating that the creation of jobs will also be encouraged, as well as the maintenance of a social organization of work in accordance with the law.The federal regulation of safety and health at work, in article 3, determines that psychosocial factors are those that cause alterations and/or disorders such as anxiety and the sleep-wake cycle as well as the presence of severe stress causing the lack of adaptation in the work environment and all the characteristics depending on the type of job you do, giving as an example the work of health professionals who come to present long and extensive working hours that are reflected thanks to various intrinsic and extrinsic factors of the person or the institution where they work. On the other hand, the Social Security Law (IMSS) mentions that if necessary, it will be the one to generate incapacity for workers, however, it does not mention that these will be given when they refer to psychosocial causes, since in the work environment these leaves will only be given without pay and with the appropriate psychological treatment to be able to overcome it. As established in Articles 41 and 43, accidents and/or illnesses caused to the person or otherwise arising as a consequence of the work environment and its characteristics, will be considered as part of the exercise of the worker's labor functions, which will be taken into account if they are included in the Federal Labor Law; Likewise, article 48 mentions that if such labor risk is caused by the employer, the institution will grant the injured party the pertinent monetary benefits, and consequently, the responsible party must reimburse the Institute for the expenses it has incurred, which is why the employer must insure the workers against labor risks that may arise in the work environment.(15)

Conclusions

The perception of the work context of health professionals in Mexico reveals a lack of appreciation, little participation in decision making and even little economic compensation, despite the constant risk to which they are exposed, regardless of the area in which they work.The COVID-19 pandemic, which originated in December 2019 in Wuhan China, affected the world as a whole and in relation to the work context of health professionals, exposed both positive and negative aspects of the various health systems. In relation to the positive aspects, it is necessary to mention the solidarity and commitment shown by all health personnel, since collaborative efforts were made to combat the situation in harmony. As for the negative aspects, in addition to the high mortality and morbidity statistics of patients and health personnel, the occupational hazards, work overload, long working hours and the physical and psychological burden that health professionals had to bear stood out(16).

Psychosocial risks, unlike psychosocial risk factors, are not organizational conditions, but rather facts, situations or states of the organism with a high probability of damaging the health of workers permanently. Psychosocial risk factors have a high probability of negatively affecting not only stress and its effects, but also detrimental damage to the worker's health, but they are avoidable, preventable conditions.Taking into account that the psychosocial origin is in the conception, organization and management of work, as well as its social and environmental context, they are manageable to reduce the potential to cause physical, social or psychological harm to workers. The probability / harm ratio of psychosocial risk factors is a function of the double gradation of the value of the probability and the severity of its consequences, which means that the psychosocial risk can range from trivial to serious and intolerable.A favorable environment must include a sense of belonging, adequate training for the performance of work activities and their clarification, proactive participation and effective communication among all members of the work team, the correct division and distribution of workloads and working hours, and their evaluation and recognition of the performance performed.Health professionals are exponentially exposed to the psychosocial risk factors that have been mentioned throughout this document, from quantitative demands, work pace, double attendance and emotional demands, which have a negative impact on their physical and mental health, as well as being reflected in the quality of activities that must be performed throughout their workday.

References

1. Orozco M, Zuluaga Y, Pulido G. Psychosocial risk factors affecting nursing professionals. Colombian Journal of Nursing [Internet]. 2019 [cited 2022 June 17];18(1). Available from: https://www.researchgate.net/publication/333862087_Factores_de_riesgo_psicosocial_que_afectan_a_los_profesionales_en_en_enfermeria.

2. Delgado-Fernández V, Rey-Merchán M del C, Arquillos AL, Delgado-Fernández V, Rey-Merchán M del C, Arquillos AL. Comparative study of occupational psychosocial risks among medical professionals. Journal of the Spanish Association of Specialists in Occupational Medicine. 2021;30(1):24-33.

3. Malacatus LAJL, Buele LARC, Romero LJAB, Choez LKDM, Malacatus LMSL, Bonoso MDGB. Psychosocial risk factors and mental health of health personnel in hospital settings. Ciencia Latina Revista Científica Multidisciplinar. on October 6, 2021;5(5):8018-35.

4. Yew SY, Yong CC, Tey NP, Cheong KC. Job satisfaction among nurses in a private hospital. International journal of health management. 2020;13:156-63.

5. Royal National Academy of Medicine: Search Engine [Internet]. [cited 2022 June 17]. Available from: https://dtme.ranm.es/buscador.aspx?NIVEL_BUS=3&LEMA_BUS=Burnout

6. Saborío Morales L, Hidalgo Murillo LF. Burnout Syndrome. Medicina Legal de Costa Rica. March 2015;32(1):119-24.

7. DOF - Official Journal of the Federation [Internet]. [cited June 17, 2022]. Available from: https://www.dof.gob.mx/nota_detalle.php?codigo=5541828&fecha=23/10/2018#gsc.tab= 0

8. 016_Dere_Labor.pdf [Internet]. [cited 2022 June 17]. Available from: https://www.gob.mx/cms/uploads/attachment/file/100174/016_Dere_Laborales.pdf

9. leyfederaldeltrabajoactualizada.pdf [Internet]. [cited 2022 June 17]. Available from: http://www.profedet.gob.mx/profedet/pdf/leyfederaldeltrabajoactualizada.pdf

10. What are Human Rights? National Human Rights Commission - Mexico [Internet]. [cited 2022 June 17]. Available from: https://www.cndh.org.mx/derechos-humanos/cuales-son-los-derechos-humanos

11. Infringement of fundamental rights at work. - Lexius Law Firm [Internet]. 2014 [cited 2022 Jun 17, 2022]. Available from: https://www.lexius.cl/articulos/derecho-del-trabajo/vulneracion-de-derechos- fundamentales-en-el-trabajo/, https://www.lexius.cl/articulos/derecho-del- trabajo/vulneracion-de-derechos-fundamentales-en-el-trabajo/.

12. Primer-DH-work.pdf [Internet]. [cited 2022 June 17]. Available from: https://www.cndh.org.mx/sites/default/files/documentos/2019-05/Cartilla-DH-trabajo.pdf

13. Quintana-Zavala MO, Bautista-Jacobo A, Velarde-Pacheco EP. Perception of the work context of nursing professionals in northwestern Mexico in times of COVID-19. SANUS. December 31, 2020;(16):1-14.

CHAPTER 9

EXPERT NURSING FUNCTIONS IN HEALTH MALPRACTICE CASES

Janet Carolina Negrón Espadas** Aurora Sierra Canto**
Omar Obeth Basto Perez* Daniela Joselin Moreno Uc* Daniela Joselin Moreno Uc*
Daniela Joselin Moreno Uc* Omar Obeth Basto Perez
The world will not be destroyed by those who do wrong, but by those who watch and do nothing.

Albert Einstein

Introduction

The main objective of health care provided by health personnel is to provide the necessary care and help restore health; these procedures must be performed with quality and professionalism in order to avoid harm to patients. However, there are a large number of cases in which mistakes are made that compromise the lives of patients and even lead to death. As a result, these malpractices lead to lawsuits by patients or their families seeking clarification and justice.It is important to mention that, in relation to this issue, in Mexico in the year 2020 the rate of cases attended at the national level per one hundred thousand inhabitants is 22.9, of which 5.0 were for non-conformities and 1.4 for complaints. Likewise, 28 awards were recorded, of which 12 had evidence of malpractice.[1]

As for the nursing expert, this is a fundamental tool in the investigation of a crime, since the expert as an expert in his field will give a perspective opinion in which he will determine if there were problems or injuries that could have been prevented.

*Student of the Bachelor's Degree in Nursing. Autonomous University of Yucatan

**Career Professor. Faculty of Nursing. Autonomous University of Yucatan

by the nursing professional who is being investigated. In nursing, the expertise is a new branch and in which there is a large field of action unknown even by nurses themselves, its importance is fundamental in cases not only of medical malpractice but also in other types of crimes in which the nurse can give his point of view based on his academic training and experience in practice.The following chapter will address the subject of nursing expertise and its role in health negligence, exposing the background of this discipline in the medical field, the regulatory framework governing the medical and nursing expertise, as well as understanding the main causes of negligence committed by health personnel and finally explaining how nursing experts participate not only in the investigation of violations of rights and mistakes by nurses towards patients, as well as its relevance in the field of hospital area. Finally, it is important to emphasize that health professionals, especially nurses, should be interested in entering the legal area, since a nursing expert will always be the most appropriate to evaluate the correct (or incorrect) actions of a colleague in a case of poor care within the health system.

Background of forensic medicine

As is well known, part of the objectives of jurists is to seek the hidden and absolute truth in the face of problems of a legal nature, and for this reason they have found it necessary to collaborate with disciplines outside their basic training that can contribute their own knowledge and thus obtain the resolution of various problems; Among these disciplines is medicine, which plays an important role as doctors are the most requested in the courts, a science that despite playing an auxiliary role within the law, has its own technical and methodological content, thus giving rise to the branch we know today as forensic medicine.[2] It is of great importance to know and approach in a general way those historical antecedents that precede the creation of forensic medicine, since according to Augusto Compte: "A science is not well known if its history is not known"; in the past the term "forensic medicine" was not known. It was not until the arrival of Numa Pompilius who began to order the physicians of that time to study the pregnant women who died, and it is here when it is thought that such actions implied expertise. It was not until the 15th century that medical-legal expertise appeared for the first time and in 1575 Ambrosio Paré published the first work on forensic medicine, giving him the title of founder of the subject. In the 16th and 17th centuries, important figures such as Orfila, Devergie Tardieu, Brouardel, Hencke, Renard, Van Hassolt, Penrose, Smith, Webster, Gromev, Pirogroff, Piaksin, Barzelloti, Lombroso, Vucetich, Lecha Marzo, appeared as the main supporters of the scientific basis of forensic medicine.[3]Regarding the historical background of forensic medicine in Mexico, it was influenced by the countries Spain, France, Germany, Italy, among others, being founded on October 23, 1833 the Establishment of Medical Sciences by decree of Don Valentin Gomez Farias President of the Mexican Republic, which also resulted in the creation of the chair of forensic medicine in 1846, and being the first director Dr. Casimiro Liceaga; He was also considered as the founder of forensic medicine in Mexico, the teacher Don Luis Hidalgo y Carpio, since he was in charge of studying everything written about forensic medicine in his time, resulting in feats such as making personal observations, being part of the commission in charge of formulating the preliminary draft of the penal code of 1871 and devising the definition that still subsists of the penal code, imposing his own broad criteria on issues of forensic medicine and writing the first work of forensic medicine together with Ruiz Sandoval in 1877.[3]

Regulatory framework for healthcare malpractice

For their part, nursing professionals are committed to act with rectitude during patient care, which is why during the exercise of their profession they must abide by the ethical and legal standards set forth at the international and national levels. Consequently, these guidelines must be known by all nursing professionals, but even more so by nursing experts since, as experts in the field, they must guide and give a fair opinion based on the law.It should be noted that at the international level there is the Universal Declaration of Human Rights of 1948, which in Article 25.1 states that "Everyone has the right to a standard of living adequate for the health and well-being of himself and his family, including food, clothing, housing, medical care and necessary social services", this right is important for health personnel because it establishes that all persons without distinction should be cared for, which is often not reflected in practice.[4] Likewise, we can count on a document for orientation and consultation of nursing professionals with a diploma or specialty in expertise (and in general of any graduate nurse or nurse in training) to the ICN (International Council of Nurses) Code of Ethics for Nurses, this guide can serve as a frame of reference for nursing practice and ethical and legal decision making.Similarly, at the national level, among the main bodies in charge of protecting the rights of patients in Mexico is the National Human Rights Commission (CNDH) with the right to health, which establishes that "every person has the right to the protection of health", as part of the fulfillment of the right to health, The General Health Law, which was published in 1984, regulates the correct care provided by doctors and nurses and allows Mexicans to have reference parameters on the obligations at the federal level and those of individuals regarding medical care, access to health services and the free exercise of the health professions.[4]

On the other hand, the National Commission for Medical Arbitration (CONAMED), created in 1996, is an institution committed to the application of conciliatory mechanisms, offering alternatives for the resolution of conflicts arising from possible negligence by health personnel in the various public and private services that make up our National Health System.[4]

On the other hand, just as there is an international code of ethics, there is the Code of Ethics for Nurses in Mexico, which regulates the conduct of nurses through moral principles, duties and obligations that guide good performance in all their professional activities.[5]

Likewise, as part of the prevention of adverse events due to negligence on the part of health personnel, there are the Essential Actions for Patient Safety, which, broadly speaking, these 8 actions are intended to improve the quality of patient care. The aim of the project is to improve service delivery, obtain and correctly record patient identification data, correct medication, improve procedural safety, reduce care-associated infection, reduce the risk of falls and record sentinel, adverse and near-miss events, as well as to measure the patient safety culture of the healthcare personnel.[6]

Finally, there is the Federal Code of Criminal Procedures, which of the list of rules presented is the most relevant or specific for medical and nursing expertise, since in its Chapter IV it establishes the requirements that professionals of any area must have to fulfill the role of expert witness and the correct way to carry out the expertise.[7]

Health negligence

In order to talk about health malpractice, it is necessary to know its origins from the approach of health services and medical care, which, although they are two similar concepts, have different definitions. According to the General Health Law, health services are "all those actions carried out for the benefit of the individual and society in general, aimed at protecting, promoting and restoring the health of the individual and the community"; likewise, medical care is defined by the General Health Law as "the set of services provided to the individual, with the purpose of protecting, promoting and restoring his health" and such activities performed by a health care provider are:[8]

• Preventive: general promotion and specific protection.

• Curative: early diagnosis and timely treatment.

• Rehabilitation: actions aimed at optimizing the capabilities and functions of people with disabilities.

• Palliative: comprehensive care to preserve the patient's quality of life through the prevention, treatment and control of pain and other physical and emotional symptoms.

However, the counterpart of adequate medical care is medical malpractice, which can be understood as the inappropriate rendering of services by medical personnel. The malpractice within the health area is characterized because such personnel acted in a negligent, imprudent or inexperienced manner, and each of these concepts has its own definitions, which are the following:[9,10]

Negligence: is the non-compliance of those principles that are known to be performed, but are still not carried out, or vice versa, it is known that they should not be performed, but the personnel continue to do so.

• Imperfection: is the lack of skills and knowledge of health personnel to carry out satisfactory and safe interventions.

Recklessness: is carrying out certain actions that are known to involve a great risk and also not taking the stipulated and necessary precautions for such interventions.

Table 1.
Examples of events that may trigger malpractice

Diagnostics	Error or delay in diagnosis. Failure to indicate relevant tests. Failure to act on the results of the tests performed Indication of inappropriate therapeutic tests. Failure to identify the patient or the diseased organ.
	Inappropriate or inadequate care. Error in the method or dosage of drug administration. Error in the administration of the treatment.

Therapeutics	Erroneous performance of surgery. Avoidable delay in treatment or response to abnormal tests. Lack of supplies and instruments. Inability to improperly perform a technique. Falsification of drugs or medications. Submission of the patient to unnecessary risk. Transgression or prohibited regulations (e.g. abortion and euthanasia not permitted by law).
Preventive	Failure to indicate prophylactic treatment. Inadequate prophylactic indications. Inadequate treatment follow-up.
	Equipment failure. Communication failure. Failure in other systems. Overconfidence, hesitancy, shyness, routine. Delays in attention. Inadequate doctor-patient relationship. Inadequate working conditions or elements. Lack of organization, discipline and supervision of the medical staff.
Others	Absence of rules for reviewing the quality of care provided. Problems in the preparation, custody and preservation of medical records. Lack of regulations governing the basic practice of the specialty. Poorly trained and poorly updated professionals. Mistreatment of the patient's family member or caregiver. Aggravation or death of the patient due to lack of quality care. Presence of unjustified injuries. Obtaining fraudulent remunerations. Presence of acts of physical and/or moral violence. Performance of medical acts without prior validation by research and/or ethics commissions and/or committees.

Taken from: Fuente-Del-Campo Antonio, Rios-Ruíz Alma. The practice of medicine and its legal environment. Cir. plást. iberolatinoam. [Internet]. 2018 [Accessed June 19, 2022]; 44 (2): 123-130. Available from: http://scielo.isciii.es/scielo.php?script=sci_arttext&pid=S0376-78922018000200002&lng=es.

Table 2.
Medical practice complaints registered in 2021 according to conamed.

Reasons for cause detailed	Sectors involved		
	Total	Public	Private
Total	2554	1423	1131
Accidents and incidents	1	0	1
Presentation of hospital-acquired infection	1	0	1
Childbirth and puerperium care	10	9	1
-Complications of childbirth	3	2	1
-Difference	5	5	0
-Lack of prenatal care	2	2	0
Diagnostic assistants	79	18	61
-Difference	44	15	29
-False positives	8	2	6
-Inopportune results	6	1	5
-Follow-up	21	0	21
Administrative and/or institutional deficiencies	15	14	1
-Prolonged delay in obtaining service	11	10	1
-Lack of medication	3	3	0
Non-medical hospital staff abuse and/or mistreatment	1	1	0
Diagnosis	936	554	382
-Difference	359	252	107
-Erroneo	167	86	81
-Lack of information and consent	308	177	131
-Unnecessary	7	0	7
-Untimely	17	11	6
-Omission	78	28	50
Physician-patient relationship	370	159	211
-Lack of information	156	72	84
-Incorrect or incomplete information	140	65	75
-Mistreatment	74	22	52
Medical treatment	882	484	398
-Premature discontinuation of treatment	2	1	1
-Secondary complications	114	45	69
-Difference	249	170	79
-Therapeutic excess	9	1	8
-Denial of service	52	29	23
-Follow-up	71	22	49
-Inadequate treatment	385	216	169
Surgical treatment	261	185	76
-Premature discharge	1	1	0
-Unnecessary surgery	3	3	0
-Postoperative complications	64	46	18

Trans-operative complications	9	4	5
-Difference of surgical treatment	94	82	12
-Follow-up	44	27	17
-Inadequate technique	37	17	20
-Lack of informed consent	1	1	0
-Lack of surveillance	8	4	4

Taken from: CONAMED. Table 7. Reasons mentioned in the presentation of concluded complaints according to detailed causes and sector of care. [PDF]. Mexico; Ministry of Health; 2021. [Accessed June 19, 2022]. Available at: https://www.gob.mx/cms/uploads/attachment/file/692290/Cuadros_Estadisticos_4oTrim_2021_07.pdf

However, so far in 2022, only the first 3 months have been recorded, with a total of 710 medical complaints concluded.[12]

Role of the nursing expert

Nurses are a fundamental pillar in the healthcare system, in the hospital environment they participate by performing acts of care always with a benevolent purpose. However, these professionals can make mistakes due to various factors during care.[13]

Now, who should judge and analyze what happened when the nursing staff commits an adverse event, would it be fair that it is evaluated by a physician or another member of the multidisciplinary team and not by another nurse? If we take into account that the expertise must be an impartial procedure and adhere to the principle of professional suitability in order to be considered an honest and fair expertise, it is logical to think that a peer professional should be the one to investigate the events that occurred since he/she could determine what the correct procedures were and point out the mistakes made by his/her colleagues.[13]

Performing an expertise among equals makes it fairer, so the nursing expertise should be performed by another nurse, and this can be supported by the medical consultation to produce a supported, not a one-sided verdict.[13]

Before delving into the role of the nursing expert witness, it is important to establish the ideal profile of an expert witness. In addition to possessing knowledge and skills in their field, they must be able to evaluate based on the healthcare context in which they find themselves, i.e., those in charge of medical care expertise must have experience at both the operational and administrative levels, as well as a broad knowledge of the care process and the legal framework that regulates all healthcare personnel.[14]

Forensic nursing and forensic nurse practitioners are still in very early stages, so there is not enough information available about their field of application at present.[15]

TABLE 3.
Forensic nursing subspecialties that go into the criminal area available in the united states and canada

Forensic Nursing Subspecialties	Description
Clinical Forensic Nurse (CFN)	Forensic nurse in charge of assisting victims of violence who are treated in the hospital setting. Responsible for documenting all information related to violence and preservation of evidence.
Forensic Nurse Investigator (FNI)	Forensic nurse working under the jurisdiction of a medical-legal office. She works in the investigation of the circumstances related to the violent act, from the circumstances of death to insurance fraud.
Forensic Nurse Examiner (FNE)	Forensic nurse who can work in various subspecialties to identify cases of interpersonal violence, especially through physical examination.
Sexual Assault Nurse Examiner (SANE)	Forensic nurse trained to act in cases of sexual violence, performing hugging, psychological support, physical examination and evidence collection.
Forensic Psychiatric Nurse Practitioner (FPN)	Forensic nurse specializing in the care of offenders with psychiatric disorders and in custody.

Taken from: Furtado Betise Mery Alencar Sousa Macau, Fernandes Carmela Lília Espósito de Alencar, Silva Juliana de Oliveira Musse, Silva Felicialle Pereira da, Esteves Rafael Braga. Research in forensic nursing: trajectories and possibilities of action. Rev. esc. enfermo USP [Internet]. 2021 [cited 2022 June 19]; 55: e20200586. Available from: http://old.scielo.br/scielo.php?script=sci_arttext&pid=S0080-62342021000100606&lng=en. Epub Sep 15, 2021.

There are also two other subspecialties that can be practiced by either forensic nurses or other types of nurses; The Nurse Consultant (LC) and the Nurse Coroner (NC) are nurses who also have training as lawyers who provide advice in cases of malpractice, negligence or any situation in which legal, civil and criminal consequences are generated, on the other hand the nurse coroner has a job closer to a medical examiner because through a specific course to be a coroner or coroner, once certified by the state these professionals can determine causes of death, assist with the identification of victims and certification of deaths of dubious cause. It is evident that North America has a long way to go when it comes to legal nursing.[15]

Table 4.
Areas of work of legal, forensic and expert nurses

No.	Work areas
1	Sexual violence.
2	Prison system.
3	Psychiatry.
4	Forensic investigation, technical assistance and consulting.
5	Evidence collection and preservation.
6	Postmortem.
7	Massive disasters, humanitarian missions and catastrophes.
8	Abuse, trauma and other forms of violence at different stages of life.

Taken from: Furtado Betise Mery Alencar Sousa Macau, Fernandes Carmela Lília Espósito de Alencar, Silva Juliana de Oliveira Musse, Silva Felicialle Pereira da, Esteves Rafael Braga. Research in forensic nursing: trajectories and possibilities of action. Rev. esc. enfermo USP [Internet]. 2021 [cited 2022 June 19]; 55: e20200586. Available from: http://old.scielo.br/scielo.php?script=sci_arttext&pid=S0080-62342021000100606&lng=en. Epub Sep 15, 2021.

Forensic nurses can act in the recognition of victims of violence, as well as elaborate individualized care plans, as well as act as court experts and based on their experience provide expert testimony.[15]

Conclusions

There is still a need for preparation in this legal area. Therefore, the search for scientific information on the subject is scarce regarding the functions of the specialist in this field. That is to say, for the purposes of this chapter, it was complex to locate references that address the role of a nursing expert at the national level, however, the educational offer of diploma courses focused on preparing human resources that address regulatory knowledge of nursing practice was identified, including health, legal and expert law, which help to soak up procedural and judicial knowledge, which are The nursing staff can be called upon in the administration of justice and act as authorized experts in the event of alleged negligence on the part of the nursing staff. Medical malpractice is the order of the day, the consequence of which is suffered by the users of health services. Being a reality the scarce preparation of nurses and expert nurses at present. After a review of the list of experts published in the year 2021 by the Judicial Power of the Federation, it was observed that only 7 are certified nursing experts, of which 4 belong to the state of Yucatan, 1 to the state of Nuevo Leon, 1 to the state of Durango and 1 to the state of Tabasco and part of Veracruz. Probably the lack of qualified nursing personnel to perform expertise functions is due to the lack of information on law at the undergraduate or graduate level, hence the need to give it the importance it needs to prepare new human resources and for nursing to excel in this area.

References

1. CAA. Platform for registration of medical complaints and opinions results 2020. [PDF]. Mexico; 2020. [Accessed June 29, 2020]. Available at: http://www.conamed.gob.mx/cmam/pdf/Resultados_Plataforma_2020_V2.pdf
2. Cartagena JM, Donat E, Barrero R, Tena E.A, Cartagena I. Manual de medicina legal para juristas. [electronic book].Santo Domingo: Editora Ortega S.R.L; 2016 [Accessed July 9, 2002]. Available at: https://www.aecid.org.do/images/noticias/Noticias/13_06_2016/DOC-20160609-WA0004.pdf.
3. Martínez, S. & Saldivar, L. Medicina Legal [PDF]. 17th ed. Mexico: Mendez Editores; 2009.
4. CONAMED. 20 años de arbitraje médico [electronic book]. Mexico: Secretaría de Salud. 2016 [Accessed June 19, 2022]. Available at: http://www.conamed.gob.mx/gobmx/libros/pdf/20anios.pdf
5. Interinstitutional Nursing Commission. Code of ethics for nurses in Mexico [electronic book]. Mexico: Secretaría de Salud 2001.
[Accessed June 19, 2022]. Available at: http://www.cpe.salud.gob.mx/site3/publicaciones/docs/codigo_etica.pdf
6. General Health Council. Acciones Esenciales Para La Seguridad del Paciente [electronic book]. Mexico: Secretaría de Salud. 2017 [Accessed June 19, 2022]. Available at: http://www.calidad.salud.gob.mx/site/calidad/docs/Acciones_Esenciales_Seguridad_Paciente.pdf.
7. Federal Code of Criminal Procedures, Official Gazette of the Federation, (Last amendment 08-20-2009)
8. General Health Law, Official Gazette of the Federation (last amendment 16-05-2021).
9. Fuente-Del-Campo Antonio, Rios-Ruíz Alma. The practice of medicine and its legal environment. Cir. plást. iberolatinoam. [Internet]. 2018 [Accessed June 19, 2022]; 44 (2): 123-130. Available from: http://scielo.isciii.es/scielo.php?script=sci_arttext&pid=S0376-78922018000200002&lng=en.
10. Vera Carrasco Oscar. HOW TO PREVENT ALLEGED MALPRACTICE SUITS MEDICAL PRAXIS. Rev Médica La Paz [Internet]. 2016 [Accessed June 19, 2022]; 22(2):60-69. Available from: http://www.scielo.org.bo/scielo.php?script=sci_arttext&pid=S1726-89582016000200011&lng=en.
11. CONAMED. Table 7. Reasons mentioned in the presentation of concluded complaints according to detailed causes and sector of care. [PDF]. Mexico; Ministry of Health; 2021. [Accessed June 19, 2022]. Available at: https://www.gob.mx/cms/uploads/attachment/file/692290/Cuadros_Estadisticos_4

oTrim_2021_07.pdf.

12. CONAMED. Table 7. Reasons mentioned in the presentation of concluded complaints according to detailed causes and sector of care. [PDF]. Mexico; Ministry of Health; 2022 [Accessed June 19, 2022]. Available at: https://www.gob.mx/cms/uploads/attachment/file/730814/Cuadro_Estadistico_07_1erTrim_2022.pdf

13. Fajardo G. Bioethical Commitment of the Nursing Expert. CONAMED Journal. Oct-Dec 2009; (144): 5-6

14. León Trejo María Enriqueta De. The expertise as an element of quality in medical care. Anest. Mex. [journal on the Internet]. 2017 [Accessed June 19, 2022]; 29(Suppl 1): 5-8. Available at: http://www.scielo.org.mx/scielo.php?script=sci_arttext&pid=S2448-87712017000400005&lng=en.

15. Furtado Betise Mery Alencar Sousa Macau, Fernandes Carmela Lília Espósito de Alencar, Silva Juliana de Oliveira Musse, Silva Felicialle Pereira da, Esteves Rafael Braga. Research in forensic nursing: trajectories and possibilities of action. Rev. esc. enfermo USP [Internet]. 2021 [cited 2022 June 19]; 55: e20200586. Available from: http://old.scielo.br/scielo.php?script=sci_arttext&pid=S0080-62342021000100006&lng=en. Epub Sep 15, 2021.

CHAPTER 10

INTERNATIONAL OCCUPATIONAL HEALTH AND SAFETY ORGANIZATIONS

Janet Carolina Negrón Espadas** Aurora Sierra Canto**
Viviana Montserrat Gallegos Mena* Lucia Jazmin Torres Montuy* Lucia Jazmin Torres Montuy* Viviana Montserrat Gallegos Mena* Lucia Jazmin Torres Montuy
"As expensive as social insurance may seem, it is less burdensome than the risks of a revolution."

Otto Von Bismark

Introduction

The actions of the government have their essential principle in the social law, since they are born with the purpose of providing solutions to the present problems of the community. In relation to health issues that are related to population growth and the emergence of diseases, it is necessary that governments create instruments and protocols for the proper use of services, thus, it is necessary that workers are aware and informed of the existence of national and international organizations in order to follow the established standards and improve the quality and safety of the worker and the company.According to the most recent global estimates, there are 2.78 million work-related deaths each year, of which 2.4 million are related to occupational diseases. In addition to the suffering this causes to workers and their families, the economic costs are enormous for companies, countries and the world in general. Losses related to compensation, lost working days, interruptions in production, training and retraining, and health care costs represent a significant proportion of the total cost of occupational diseases.

*Student of the Bachelor's Degree in Nursing. Autonomous University of Yucatan

**Career Professor. Faculty of Nursing. Autonomous University of Yucatan about 3.94 percent of GDP. For employers, this translates into costly early retirements, loss of qualified personnel, absenteeism and high insurance premiums. However, these situations could be avoided by acquiring rational methods of prevention, reporting and inspection that, through the occupational safety and health agencies provided to governments, employers and workers for the purpose of developing the necessary tools to ensure maximum safety at work.In this chapter, the main national and international organizations that provide the worker, employer and company with information, principles, standards and requirements to promote occupational health at work will be discussed in general terms.

International Organizations

As mentioned above, several international organizations that focus on the health of the working population will be presented: The World Health Organization, the International Labor Organization, the International Social Security Association, the American Conference of Governmental Industrial Hygienists, the International Agency for Research on Cancer, the National Institute for Occupational Safety and

Health, the Ibero-American Social Security Organization, the Occupational Safety and Health Administration, the American Industrial Hygiene Association, the National Center for Occupational Health and Safety Information Security, the Occupational Health and Safety Assessment Series, and the International Organization for Standardization. [1]

World Health Organization

Its main objective is to build a better and healthier world for people around the world through the slogan "Improving health for all". It was inaugurated on April 7, 1948, the same day that World Health Day is celebrated. The WHO is a directive and coordinating authority on international health situations. Among the activities it carries out are the search for communicable and non-communicable diseases, surveillance and control of health crises, and health promotion in different areas of the life cycle through international health systems and services. [2]

It also provides technical cooperation to members around the world to support the development and continuous improvement of safe and healthy workplaces. It therefore liaises with a variety of stakeholders from different occupational sectors to effectively prevent illness, injury and death in the work environment, as well as to respond to global, regional and national priorities in occupational safety and health. [2]

International Labor Organization

The International Labor Organization (ILO) aims to promote labor rights, principles and standards, manage decent work opportunities, enhance social security, and strengthen effective, tripartite communication in addressing labor-related issues. [3]

The present organization brings together governments, employers and workers from 187 member states for the purpose of enacting labor regulations and standards, proposing policies and developing programs to promote decent work for all, women and men. It also establishes that workers and employers have the same rights as governments through the discussions of the ILO's main bodies due to its tripartite nature, and guarantees that their opinions are expressed in its standards, policies and programs. It also defends the protection of social justice, universal human and labor rights, claiming social justice as the main link to global and definitive peace. [3]

It also carries out its work through three fundamental bodies: the International Labor Conference, which sets universal labor standards and determines the general policies of the Organization, the Governing Body, which is the governing body that makes decisions, and the International Labor Office, which is basically the permanent advisory office responsible for supervisory activities. [3]

International Social Security Association

The world's leading social security organization is the International Social Security Association (ISSA), which was inaugurated in 1927 under the auspices of the ILO. The ISSA brings together social security institutions, ministries and government agencies to maintain excellence in social security administration through professional standards, social security expertise, services and expert support in shaping dynamic policies and systems around the world. [4]

Among the activities carried out by this organization are the creation of standards, research and analysis for the selection of good practices, providing data on security systems in a total of 177 countries, as well as providing practical support services to social security administrations; it promotes new approaches to achieve better administration by anticipating possible risks and, if necessary, making the appropriate changes. [4]

American Conference of Governmental Industrial Hygienist

The ACGIH is a scientific charitable corporation that is directed to those professionals involved in occupational health, environmental, safety and, as its name implies, industrial hygiene. Notably, this organization is comprised of a board of directors and committees, organized by members who seek to provide critical and current information to government, academia and corporate facilities throughout the United States, Canada and countries abroad. [5]

Some of the information provided by ACGIH is based primarily on topics related to industrial hygiene, which relates to risk control, identification and creation of protocols that anticipate and evaluate actions that may endanger worker health and well-being, environmental health and health safety issues through courses, forums, downloadable resources and conferences. [5]

International Agency for Research on Cancer

The International Agency for Research on Cancer (IARC) was created on May 20, 1965 as a result of an initiative of a group of French public figures whose objectives were to reduce the increasing burden of cancer in the world's population. humanity. Its headquarters building is located in Lyon, France, but it now has offices in a total of 26 countries. [6]

The IARC is a specialized cancer organization, which belongs to the WHO. Its main objective is to achieve international collaboration on cancer research. It is responsible for identifying the causes of cancer in order to implement preventive measures to reduce the burden of disease and associated suffering. It coordinates research with countries and organizations, especially those in low- and middle-income countries. [6]

It cooperates in terms of reducing tobacco consumption, implementing vaccination against viruses associated with the cause of cancer or evaluating the effectiveness of intervention strategies. This organization does not participate directly in the implementation of control measures, nor does it carry out research on the treatment or care of cancer patients; however, all the recommendations made by this organization help to prevent accidents or occupational diseases, thus achieving greater safety and health in the workplace. [6]

National Institute for Occupational Safety and Health

The National Institute for Occupational Safety and Health (NIOSH) is the federal agency that commissions the production of research and suggestions for the prevention of occupational illnesses and injuries. [7]

At the same time, it aims to provide current knowledge in the area of occupational health and safety in order to adapt that information to the practice to promote the progress of employees. To achieve its objective, NIOSH conducts scientific research, produces mandatory standards and recommendations, issues warnings and analyzes occupational hazards through a systematized evaluation. [7]

This organization provides national and international leadership to prevent illness, injury or occupational hazards that may lead to employee disability or death. This is done through data collection, scientific research and the use of knowledge. [7]

Ibero-American Social Security Organization

The OISS, which stands for "Organización Iberoamericana de Seguridad Social", is a specialized international organization with a technical character, whose objective is to promote the economic and social welfare of the Ibero-American countries and those united by the Spanish and Portuguese languages through the coordination, exchange and use of their mutual experiences in Social Security and in the field of social protection. [8]

As stated above, the OISS is responsible for responding to existing needs in the field of Social Security, as well as providing close and effective collaboration between the institutions that confirm it. [8]

The services offered include human resources training, cooperation, assistance and technical support for the modernization of the management of the Social Security Systems, programs to promote the development of social security in Ibero-America, study, debate and research activities and activities of statutory and community bodies, relations with other national and international organizations, information and dissemination activities. [8]

Occupational Safety and Health Administration

The Occupational Safety and Health Administration (OSHA) is part of the U.S. Department of Labor and seeks the circumstances and work requirements that lead to adequate employee health and safety. It also promotes compliance with regulations and provides worker training, education, and assistance. [9]

Through this organization, you can find different topics related to workers' rights, preventive actions to avoid the risk of falls, personal protective equipment and different issues that provide assistance to the employee and employer. It also offers resources and applications to file a complaint, prevent suicide, provides web pages on its platform on safety and health issues and training in this area.[9]

American Industrial Hygiene Association

The American Industrial Hygiene Association (AIHA) is one of the largest international associations focused on serving occupational and environmental health needs. Its purpose is to help occupational and environmental health and safety hazards to be anticipated and eliminated or, conversely, controlled. This association is charged with the promotion of the profession and the practice of occupational and environmental health and safety hazards in industry, government and society, and seeks to improve the practice of occupational and environmental health and safety hazards and the knowledge and competence of professionals; it also provides a global forum for the exchange of information and ideas regarding occupational and environmental health and safety hazards and, finally, it seeks to represent the profession nationally and internationally.[10] The mission is to empower and promote those who apply scientific knowledge to protect all workers and their communities from occupational and environmental hazards. [10]

National Centre for Occupational Health and Safety Information

The National Center for Occupational Health and Safety Information, acronym CCOHS, offers a variety of documents and reports related to laws and regulations, health and safety programs, and worker rights and responsibilities. Through these topics, it promotes training and summaries on the handling and transportation of dangerous goods, chemical, ergonomic, physical, psychosocial and biological hazards and risks, as well as safety issues and exposure to unhealthy and substandard workplaces. [11] In addition, through this body, safe work activities and procedures are managed, with health promotion initiatives and risk assessments according to the age of the employee. [11] In conclusion, the variety of programs offered by this center is broad, ranging from hazard identification, risk assessment, emergency response, and emergency preparedness and response. accident investigations to safety and health committees, violence prevention and workplace inspections. [11]

Occupational Health and Safety Assessment Series

OHSAS, in Spanish "Sistemas de Gestión de Seguridad y Salud en el Trabajo", provides a series of requirements for occupational health and safety management systems allowing organizations to manage their risks and improve their work performance. These management systems can be applied in organizations that wish to establish guidelines to eliminate or minimize the risk of employees being exposed to occupational safety and health risks associated with their work activities, also for those who want to implement, maintain and improve their occupational safety and health management, those organizations seeking certification/registration of their occupational safety and health management system by an external organization. [12]

Its motto is: "Continuous improvement" which is structured by a series of key points that are simplified in: planning, implementation and operation, verification and corrective action, management review and finally, the implementation of the safety and health policy at work. [13]

International Organization for Standardization

The International Organization for Standardization is an autonomous non-governmental organization with 167 national bodies. With regard to its members, it groups experts, who, in turn, collaborate and distribute knowledge in order to promote voluntary International Standards based on agreements and approvals of the participating personnel for the benefit of the employee, promoting innovation and results to the universal labor challenges. All this is due to the fact that every day workers die due to work-related accidents or illnesses and this organization aims to help agencies prevent accidents and illnesses of this origin, managing through a framework of reference those risks and opportunities for safety and health at work. [14]

The development of international standards is intended to provide the employee and employer with certainty of safety, quality and reliability. Through the facilitation of employee training and assistance programs, it is intended to fulfill part of the United Nations Sustainable Development Goals by increasing the benefits of international standardization and supporting the adoption of ISO Standards. [14]

National Organizations

The following is a description of the national organizations responsible for occupational health: the Political Constitution of the United Mexican States, the Federal Labor Law and the Federal Regulations on Occupational Safety and Health. [1]

Political Constitution of the United Mexican States

Occupational safety and health is regulated by several precepts contained in the Constitution. This is the most important document in the country and it stipulates the foundations to ensure fairness in the administration of justice in all senses, among them, that which refers to occupational safety and health, which is supported by the corresponding laws, which in turn are structured based on international conventions, which are considered supreme law. In its sixth title, "Labor and Social Welfare", Article 123, which states "Every person has the right to decent and socially useful work; to this end, the creation of jobs and the social organization of work will be promoted, in accordance with the law", mentions the rights and obligations of workers and employers. [15]

Federal Labor Law

The Federal Labor Law is the highest document of labor law in Mexico and only the Mexican Constitution is above it. The labor rules seek to achieve stability among the agents of production and social justice, as well as to favor a dignified work environment. This law contains the rights and obligations of workers and employers, where the causes or reasons for termination of the contract, the obligations of the worker, the types of disability caused by work-related illnesses and the rights that a worker acquires as a result of a work-related illness or accident are set forth. This The purpose of this document is to provide the worker with a dignified or decent job where full respect for human dignity is a priority; through the sole existence of equality and with the obligation of access to social security, beneficial salary, with continuous training for the enhancement of productivity and with the existence of optimal conditions of safety and hygiene to prevent occupational hazards. [16]

Federal Regulation on Occupational Safety and Health

The purpose of this regulation is to implement the provisions on Occupational Safety and Health that must be present in the Work Centers, in order to have the conditions to prevent risks and thus guarantee workers the right to perform their activities in environments that ensure their life and health, based on the provisions of the Federal Labor Law. It comes into force on February 13, 2015 and is addressed to employers, employees and competent authorities. [17]

This document contains all the competencies, obligations, administrative sanctions, occupational health and safety standards, general provisions, special occupational health and safety precautions, occupational accidents and diseases, support to facilitate knowledge and compliance with regulations, consultation mechanisms and the monitoring and verification of compliance with regulations. [17]

Conclusion

Companies and states usually talk about occupational safety when they talk about high costs, however, they do not take into account the enormous economic risks posed by hazardous conditions and unsafe acts that are caused by occupational hazards and the effects on workers' health.Approximately 65% of the Region's population is in the labor force, and the average worker spends about two-thirds of his or her life at work. Work is not only a source of income, but also a fundamental element of health, status, social relations, and life opportunities. Compared to the international level, in the country there are few organizations or documents that protect the health of workers or that provide relevant information for risk prevention. That is why these international organizations are so important, because through their standards, protocols, research and documents, they provide workers with the information necessary to know their rights and obligations. It is considered that at the national level more organizations should be implemented in which both employees and employers can support each other; on the other hand, it is of utmost importance that the target population knows about these organizations created for their help and care during their work performance. Although workers have rights established in national documents, they are violated by ignorance of their presence.From the human point of view, workers are not tools of labor, but the living force that keeps a company or a nation afloat. What Otto Von Bismark pointed out in the 19th century when he uttered the phrase: "However expensive social security may seem, it is cheaper than a social revolution" was a reference to the threats that the State may face when workers rise up against an oppressive State. These same ideas are applied to companies that, ignoring the value of workers as the driving force of the business, consider as an expense anything that is done for the benefit of their safety; however, the costs established by the Federal Labor Law in the event of a labor risk are so great that they can lead to the bankruptcy of a company. That is why there are organizations that promote actions for the benefit of the worker and the company, preventing risks, violence and accidents at work.

References

1. Mexican Institute of Social Security. National and International Regulations on the Prevention of Occupational Risks. Mexico. 2022.
2. World Health Organization. About WHO; Who we are. [Internet] [Internet

[Cited June 15, 2022] Available at: https://www.who.int/es/about/who- we-are

3. International Labor Organization. About the ILO. [Internet] [Cited 17 June 2022]. Available from: https://www.ilo.org/global/about-the-ilo/lang-- en/index.htm.
4. International Social Security Association. About ISSA. [Internet] [Cited June 16, 2022] Available at: https://ww1.issa.int/es/about/the- issa.
5. ACGIH. Defining Science for OEHS Experts. About ACGIH. [Internet] [Cited July 17, 2022]. Available from: https://www.acgih.org/about/about-us/
6. International Agency for Research on Cancer. About IARC [Internet] [Accessed June 16, 2022] Available at: https://www.iarc.who.int/cards_page/about-iarc/
7. CDC. Centers for Disease Control and Prevention. National Institute for Occupational Safety and Health (NIOSH). About NIOSH. [Internet] [Cited June 17, 2022]. Available at: https://www.cdc.gov/spanish/niosh/ab-sp.html
8. Ibero-American Social Security Organization. The OISS. [Internet] [Cited June 16, 2022] Available at: https://oiss.org/que-es-la-oiss/
9. United States Department Of Labor. Occupational Safety and Health Administration. [Internet[[Cited June 16, 2022]. Available from: I am OSHA | Occupational Safety and Health Administration.
10. American Industrial Hygiene Association (AIHA). About AIHA. [Internet] 2022. [Cited June 16, 2022] Available at: https://www.aiha.org/about-aiha.
11. CCOHS. Canadian Centre for Occupational Health and Safety. About CCOHS. [Internet] [Cited June 17, 2022]. Available from: CCOHS: Projects and Partnerships.
12. Canadian Center for Occupational Health and Safety. OHSAS 18001. Canada. [Internet] 2022 [Cited June 16, 2022] Available at: https://www.ccohs.ca/products/oshworks/ohsas18001.html
13. A, Perales. Implementation of a health and safety management system based on

the OHSAS 18001 standard. Polytechnic University of Catalonia. Barcelona. [Internet] 2017. [Cited June 16, 2022] Available at:

https://upcommons.upc.edu/bitstream/handle/2117/108636/Mem%C3%B2ria_Per alesAntoni.pdf?sequence=1&isAllowed=y

14. ISO. What we do. Capacity building. [Internet] [Cited June 17, 2022]. Available at: https://www.iso.org/capacity-building.html

15. Secretary of Parliamentary Services. Political Constitution of the United Mexican States. Official Gazette of the Federation. Mexico [Internet] 2021. [Last accessed on June 16, 2022] Available at:

https://www.diputados.gob.mx/LeyesBiblio/pdf/CPEUM.pdf

16. Chamber of Deputies of the H. Congress of the Union. Federal Labor Law. Last Reform DOF 18-05-2022. [Internet] [Cited June 17, 2022]. Available at: https://www.diputados.gob.mx/LeyesBiblio/pdf/LFT.pdf

17. Secretary of Labor and Social Welfare. Federal Regulation on Occupational Safety and Health. Official Gazette of the Federation. Mexico. [Internet] 2014 [Cited June 16, 2022] Available at: http://asinom.stps.gob.mx:8145/upload/RFSHMAT.pdf

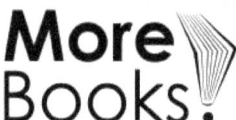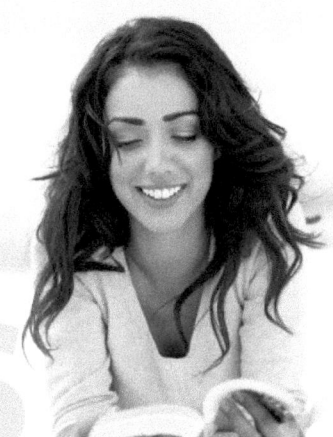

I want morebooks!

Buy your books fast and straightforward online - at one of world's fastest growing online book stores! Environmentally sound due to Print-on-Demand technologies.

Buy your books online at
www.morebooks.shop

Kaufen Sie Ihre Bücher schnell und unkompliziert online – auf einer der am schnellsten wachsenden Buchhandelsplattformen weltweit! Dank Print-On-Demand umwelt- und ressourcenschonend produzi ert.

Bücher schneller online kaufen
www.morebooks.shop

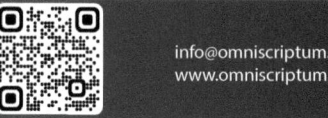
info@omniscriptum.com
www.omniscriptum.com
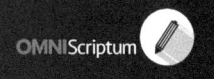

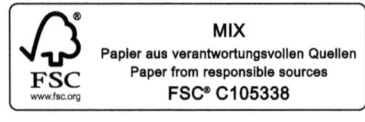

Printed by Books on Demand GmbH, Norderstedt / Germany